HOW TO GROW

MEDICINAL HERBS

An Illustrated Beginner's Guide to Growing, Harvesting, and Making Herbal Remedies at Home

VANESSA MINTON
Creator of From the Garden

ADAMS MEDIA

NEW YORK   AMSTERDAM/ANTWERP   LONDON   TORONTO   SYDNEY/MELBOURNE   NEW DELHI

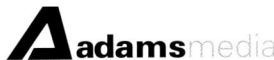

Adams Media
An Imprint of Simon & Schuster, LLC
100 Technology Center Drive
Stoughton, MA 02072

First Adams Media hardcover edition June 2026

ADAMS MEDIA and colophon are registered trademarks of Simon & Schuster, LLC.

Simon & Schuster strongly believes in freedom of expression and stands against censorship in all its forms. For more information, visit BooksBelong.com.

For information about special discounts for bulk purchases, please contact Simon & Schuster Special Sales at 1-866-506-1949 or business@simonandschuster.com.

The Simon & Schuster Speakers Bureau can bring authors to your live event. For more information or to book an event, contact the Simon & Schuster Speakers Bureau at 1-866-248-3049 or visit our website at www.simonspeakers.com.

Interior design by Sylvia McArdle
Illustrations by Brynn Wilcox, Swashy Studio

Manufactured in China

10 9 8 7 6 5 4 3 2 1

Library of Congress Control Number: 2025949139

ISBN 978-1-5072-2599-8
ISBN 978-1-5072-2600-1 (ebook)

Many of the designations used by manufacturers and sellers to distinguish their products are claimed as trademarks. Where those designations appear in this book and Simon & Schuster, LLC, was aware of a trademark claim, the designations have been printed with initial capital letters.

This book is intended as general information only and should not be used to diagnose or treat any health condition. In light of the complex, individual, and specific nature of health problems, this book is not intended to replace professional medical advice. The ideas, procedures, and suggestions in this book are intended to supplement, not replace, the advice of a trained medical professional. Consult your physician before adopting any of the suggestions in this book, as well as about any condition that may require diagnosis or medical attention. The author and publisher disclaim any liability arising directly or indirectly from the use of this book.

This book is dedicated to my children, Evelyn, Oliver, and Troy, who brought me into motherhood...an experience that led me to herbalism in more ways than one. From teas that helped me heal from giving birth, to boosting my milk supply, and sensitive skin–safe healing salves for the inevitable bruises and scrapes of childhood, I've found myself more often in the garden, leaning on my herbal companions to help heal my family throughout the years.

They are the inspiration for my never-ending pursuit of knowledge, growth, and healing, and the foundation for the advice that I share in this guide.

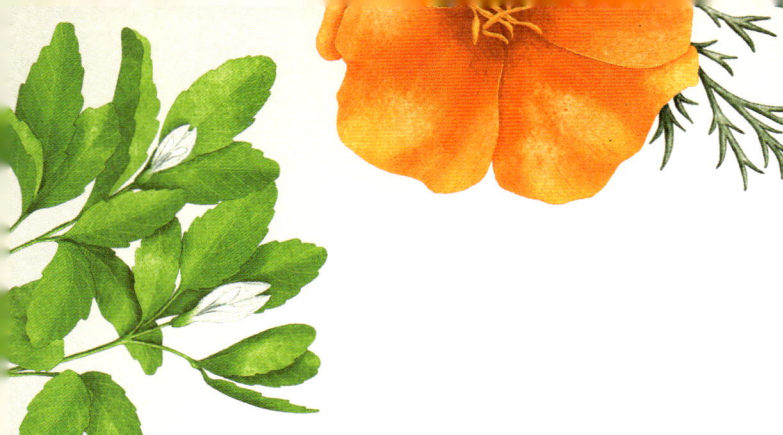
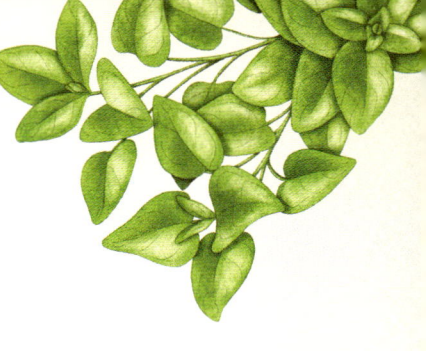

Contents

PART 1

Getting Started   8

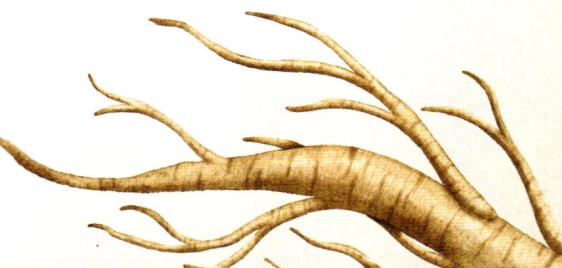

Making Tinctures and Salves 26

Adding Herbs to Meals and Drinks   43

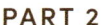

PART 2

Medicinal Herbs   63

Terms to Know . . . 64

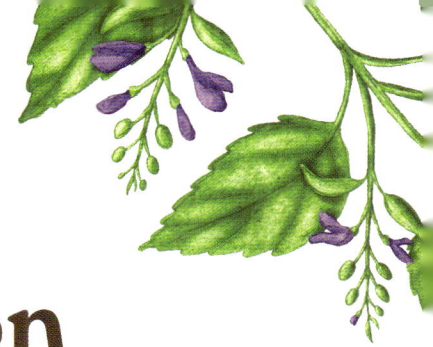

Introduction

Ginger for digestive relief. Echinacea for immune support. Calendula for wound healing. Passion vine to ease anxiety. You can grow these and dozens more herbs in your own home or garden for all-natural health benefits.

Starting your own medicinal herb garden is easier than you think. In fact, growing herbs is perfect for beginners and longtime gardeners alike. Most can be grown in small spaces or pots and are resilient, fragrant, and as lovely as they are useful. Whether you're planting your first mint sprig or dreaming of a full backyard apothecary, this book will teach you everything you need to know to grow herbs for medicinal use. You'll learn how to:

- Plan what you'll grow based on your location and space.
- Determine the differences between annuals and perennials and woody and herbaceous herbs.
- Decide whether seeds or seedlings are a better choice.
- Manage unwanted garden pests.

Your garden can feature either specific herbs for your personal needs or a wide range of plants that offer a myriad of benefits. To give you inspiration, each of the fifty beautifully illustrated herb profiles provides a comprehensive overview of everything you need to know about that plant, from its topical and internal uses to unique varieties and specific growing tips.

Once your plants are growing, you'll also discover exactly how to preserve and transform your thriving herbs into simple, effective remedies. After you learn which simple tools you'll need and how to dry herbs for storage without losing their potency, you can begin crafting personalized treatments, from teas and infusions to tinctures and salves. You'll find simple and effective ways to address common concerns like rashes, pain and inflammation, nausea, headaches, and immune system functioning.

Growing medicinal herbs isn't just about filling your medicine cabinet with natural remedies. You'll also develop a strong connection to your garden, including its fragrances and tastes, as well as the care each plant needs to thrive. Your body and mind will thrive as well—one leaf, one sip, and one remedy at a time.

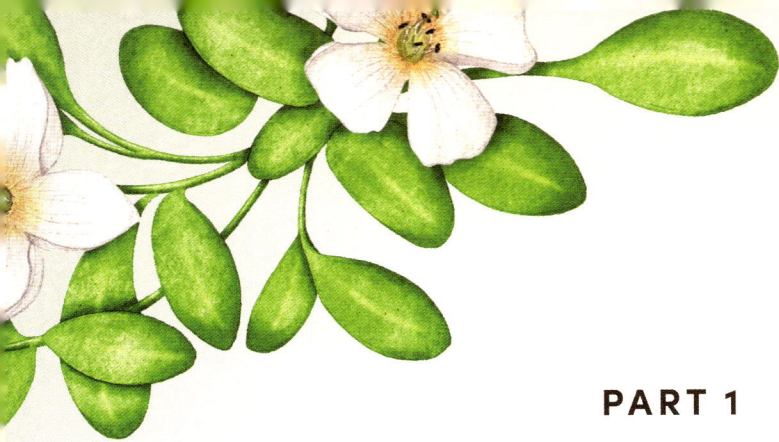

PART 1

Getting Started

The chapters in this part will walk you through the entire process of starting a medicinal herb garden. You'll learn important foundational gardening information in Chapter 1, like hardiness zones and growing season length, which will help you know which plants could grow well in your area. After you gain an understanding of the various types of herbs and plants in your garden, you'll learn how to deal with pests and how to properly prune your plants. Once your plants are growing, Chapter 2 will show you how to use them to soothe your body and mind.

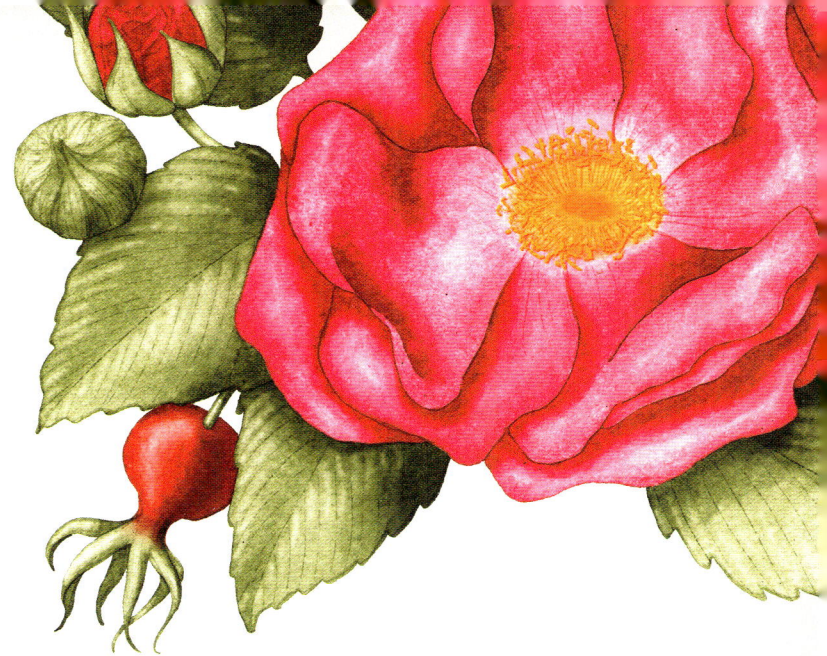

You'll learn the proper way to harvest leaves, flowers, and roots; find a list of the simple tools you'll need to work with them; and get guidance for using them to create infused teas and oils, salves, glycerites, tinctures, poultices, and more. Chapter 3 highlights the culinary value of these healing herbs with several recipes featuring delicious foods that can also improve your health. By the end of this part, you'll be able to plant, harvest, and utilize your medicinal herb garden.

CHAPTER 1

The Basics of Growing a Medicinal Herb Garden

This chapter will walk you through the essential knowledge every beginner needs to get started: understanding how different types of herbs grow, learning your climate, choosing the right location for planting, understanding soil and water needs, selecting containers or garden beds, and creating the conditions for long-term success. If you already consider yourself to be an established gardener, this will be a great refresher on plant-growing information with a focus on medicinal herb cultivation. If you've never grown a plant successfully, this chapter will demystify the wonderful world of garden planning, maintenance, harvesting, and plant life cycles. This is the foundation you will build your herbal practice upon to take you from your first seeds to a full medicine cabinet of homegrown remedies!

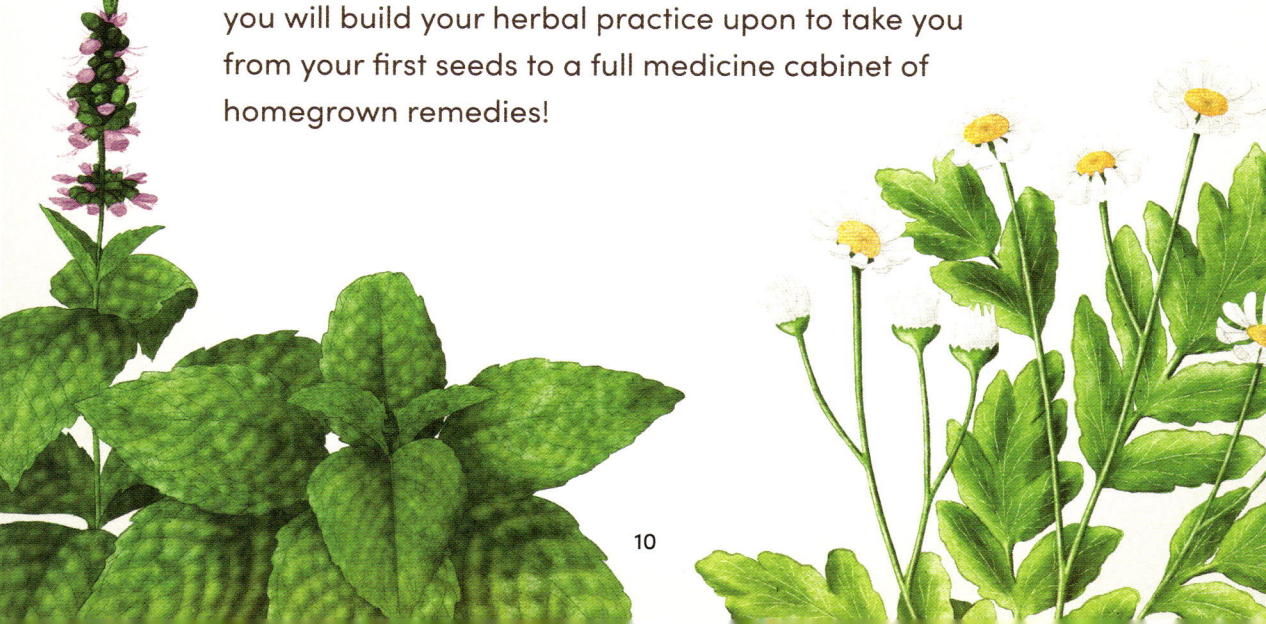

Understanding USDA Growing Zones

Before you start planting, it's essential to know two key things about your location: your USDA hardiness zone and your growing season length. These will help you know which types of herbs will survive your local climate and when to plant them.

The USDA Plant Hardiness Zone Map (available at https://planthardiness.ars.usda.gov, and searchable by zip code) divides the United States into thirteen zones, with the low-numbered zones being the coldest and the high-numbered zones being the warmest. These zone temperature calculations are based on the average annual minimum winter temperatures recorded—*not* the average winter temperature and *not* the coldest it's ever been in your area. The zones are made using the coldest temperature that typically happens once per year on average over a rolling 30-year cycle. This average is updated every decade, which means that your zone can change. With recent warmer average winter temperatures for the majority of North America, many gardeners' zones shifted one subzone warmer recently as the 30-year average was recalculated in 2023.

Each zone represents a 10°F temperature range, and every zone is then broken up into A and B subzones with 5°F differences. For example, zone 8a lists temps at 10–15°F and 8b lists temps at 15–20°F. To find your zone, visit the website and enter your zip code.

It's important to note that zone temperatures are a long-term *average*, not a guarantee. Your zone might be zone 8b (15–20°F) but it's still possible to have an occasional 10°F night. Always assume your garden could dip at least ten degrees colder than your zone suggests at least once per winter.

GROWING ZONE LIMITATIONS

Growing zones are based on cold tolerance, not summer heat. But heat can also have a significant effect on plants: Some herbs may tolerate frost but collapse in extreme heat. If you garden in a hot area, it's just as important to understand:

- How hot your summers get.
- How long extreme heat typically lasts.
- How much annual rainfall you get, along with the average daily humidity levels.

Connect with local gardeners or Cooperative Extensions to learn what has worked well for them. (Coop Extensions, often called "local ag extensions," are county-based offices that share research-based information on agriculture, gardening, nutrition, and natural resources. Nearly every US county has an extension office.)

How to Calculate Your Growing Season

Finding the average frost dates for your area can help you understand when your growing season starts and ends each year. Your growing season is the number of frost-free days between your last frost (32°F) in the spring and your first frost in the fall/winter. For example, if your last frost is April 15 and your first frost is October 20, your growing season is 188 days long.

You can find out the average calculated frost dates for your area by going to https://almanac.com/gardening/frostdates and entering your zip code. This information can help you plan for planting and harvesting herbs like basil, which won't survive a frost, and it gives you a deadline for harvesting usable plant growth from herbs that can survive a frost but may drop their leaves and flowers during winter months. Remember that the average frost date information is just that—an *average* based on your general area. Once you start gardening, you should keep notes on your own observed frost dates and plant survival to build a personalized planting calendar over time for your specific garden.

Perennial versus Annual Herbs

To understand how herbs grow, you'll need to know the difference between the two main types of herb lifespans that exist: perennial and annual herbs.

- **Perennial herbs** live for multiple years, regrowing each spring from the same root system. In colder climates, they may die back in winter, but they should return when the weather warms. They're great "anchor" plants for your herb garden and require less replanting. For most perennial herbs, the winter season will cause the plants to look as if they have died completely.

But if their root systems remain healthy and intact, the chances are good that they will remerge in the spring. This process is called "dormancy." However, some perennials can maintain a living appearance throughout the colder months. These types of plants are called "evergreens" due to the plant's ability to stay forever green.
- **Biennial herbs** are a less common type of short-lived perennial that put on most of their leafy, above-ground growth in their first year of life and send up a flower stalk in their second year of life that eventually produces seeds for reproduction purposes. This type of plant will then die completely after its 2-year life cycle has finished with the production of seeds.
- **Annual herbs** complete their life cycle in one season. They will die completely with the first actual frost of the winter season, typically in late fall. This means you'll need to replant them annually each spring. These fast growers can be tucked into open spaces around perennials for seasonal harvests.

An important note: Some herbs behave differently depending on where you live. An herb like rosemary is a perennial in warmer zones (8–10) but may need protection or replanting in colder zones (3–7). A diverse yet manageable herb garden mixes perennials for structure and annuals for variety. What this mix actually looks like for *you* will depend on your climate, desired goals, space, and available resources.

Identifying Types of Herbs

The next step in developing the plant list for your medicinal herb garden is to understand how herbs can be classified by their stems, root behavior, and growth habits. These traits affect how much space they need, how hardy they are, and where they'll thrive in your garden design.

STEM TYPES

At the simplest level, herbs can be divided into two stem categories: woody-stemmed and shrublike or herbaceous and tender-stemmed. Knowing which type you're planting helps you match the herb to the right location. For example, woody-stemmed herbs tolerate drought well, so they're perfect for hot, dry areas of the garden that don't receive frequent watering. Herbaceous, tender-stemmed herbs need more consistent care and moisture, so they do better near pathways, in lower-lying garden spots, or in a place where they'll get frequent attention.

Woody-Stemmed Herbs

Woody herbs develop tough, bark-like stems and become similar to shrubs over time. New green growth emerges each season, while the base becomes permanent and woody. In warm climates, they can remain evergreen. In colder climates, tender growth may die back each winter, but the woody base structure supports regrowth in spring. They are generally long-lived perennials that benefit from light pruning to maintain shape. Examples include rosemary, lavender, thyme, oregano, and sage.

Herbaceous, Tender-Stemmed Herbs

Herbaceous herbs have fully green, flexible stems that usually die back completely at the first frost. Many are fast-growing annuals or tender perennials, surviving winter only in frost-free climates. Examples include basil, cilantro, and roselle hibiscus. They usually require regular pruning or pinching to help prevent bolting and extend your harvest, and they either reseed naturally or need annual replanting.

VISUAL GROWTH TYPES

In addition to stem hardiness type, herbs can grow in different ways that affect the space they take up in the garden:

- **Upright growers:** Echinacea, roselle hibiscus, and marshmallow need vertical space and may form stalks or clumps that shoot up flowering stems.
- **Creeping or spreading herbs:** Mint, lemon balm, and catnip grow outward along the ground or through underground runners.
- **Tall and airy:** Yarrow, chamomile, and feverfew grow tall, with umbrella-shaped flower clusters and wispy leaves.

Consider planting vertical growers along the back side of garden beds while mixing in low-growing, spreading herbs in front or near pathways to give breathing room and visual appeal to your garden.

HERB ROOT TYPES

Some medicinal herbs grow deep taproots, which allow them to draw minerals from layers far below the surface. Others spread quickly through underground stems or roots, which can make them aggressive in the garden. Understanding these root growth habits will help you decide whether to give an herb a permanent spot in the ground or keep it contained in a bed or pot.

Taproot Herbs

Certain medicinal herbs develop a strong taproot. They usually have a single, sturdy root, sometimes with two to three main branches that grow deep into the soil. These herbs are sometimes called dynamic accumulators because they pull micronutrients and minerals from the soil and concentrate them in their leaves and roots.

Taproot herbs are often long-lived perennials and may be dug up partially for root harvesting and drying for medicinal use. They don't always transplant well or flourish in shallow containers because of this singular root system. They can withstand dry spells because of their access to deep water reserves, and they're frequently long-lived, returning year after year. Examples of taprooted herbs include dandelion, valerian, echinacea, and comfrey.

Aggressive Spreaders

Many herbs in the mint family (Lamiaceae), such as mint, oregano, thyme, catnip, and lemon balm, spread by underground rhizomes and runners. A rhizome is a type of underground stem that grows horizontally through the soil. These herbs can quickly take over garden beds if left unchecked thanks to their "runners" forming underground colonies. They are easy to propagate, but they often do best when contained in pots, raised beds, or dedicated areas where spreading is welcome. Spreading herbs often have desirable, fragrant foliage, but be wary of their invasive nature.

Soil Requirements

Different herbs have different soil needs depending on how they grow and the type of container or garden bed they are grown in. These needs primarily come down to the type of water drainage each herb prefers.

SOIL NEEDS FOR DIFFERENT TYPES OF HERBS

- **Woody-stemmed herbs** need excellent drainage and do well in sandy soil or cactus soil (premixed, fast-draining soil blends that have low organic matter and higher amounts of chunky materials) for container growing. The biggest risk for woody-stemmed herbs is rotting at the top of the woody root. They actually prefer "poor" soil and don't need much compost or fertilizer. For planting these herbs in the ground, consider higher areas of your garden that receive full sun (even in the South). For container growing these herbs, grow bags and terracotta pots are a great option, as their porous nature boosts drainage.

- **Herbaceous, tender-stemmed herbs and spreaders,** like mint, prefer soil that holds moisture. For planting in containers or raised beds, you can use a basic store-bought potting mix or a DIY potting mix of one-third coconut coir (the dried shredded husk of the coconut that holds water well), one-third compost, and one-third vermiculite (a naturally occurring mineral that expands into spongy flakes that retain moisture while slowly releasing it to to surrounding soil as needed). This ratio was originally created by Square Foot Gardening creator Mel Bartholomew to help retain moisture while gently feeding your plants. To plant these herbs in the ground, you can amend native soil (the natural, original soil found in the ground) by mixing in compost to the planned garden area. Some native soil may be a hard clay texture, so opting for laying compost on top of this soil will help it soften and increase drainage over time.
- **Taprooted/accumulator herbs** can tolerate a variance in soil quality, as long as they have access to a water source. Their ability to survive in drought conditions and poor soil is due to their ability to send down a long root to access deeper water reserves. If they aren't given this access, you will need to support their moisture needs by supplementing periods of drought with manual waterings. This is more of a concern when growing taprooted herbs in containers, as they can dry out quicker, and containers do not allow them to grow to their full potential. The smaller the container you grow them in, the more you will need to focus on keeping the soil consistently moist. If grown in a raised garden bed, you should opt for one with an open bottom to allow the taproot to grow deep and access nutrients in the soil.

HOW TO TEST SOIL DRAINAGE PROPERTIES

You can test your soil's drainage by watering it thoroughly. If water soaks into the soil but seems to pool and flood the area for more than 20 seconds, you may need to add compost, perlite (a lightweight porous material made from volcanic glass that adds aeration to increase drainage), or sand to improve drainage. But never add sand to clay soil, as it can harden like concrete!

If the soil stays dry underneath while water sits on top, it may be hydrophobic (soil that repels water instead of absorbing it). This is usually a symptom of soil that has been allowed to get very dry for a period of time. Try using warm water to help it absorb moisture, or add 1 teaspoon of castile soap to a 1-gallon watering can for a single watering to break the surface tension and allow water to penetrate down. Or, manually push a stick into the soil every few inches, being mindful not to damage roots, and fill those holes with water to allow the moisture to soak in deeper.

To help soil retain moisture between waterings, consider covering the soil in your containers and garden beds with 2–4" of one of these options: chopped straw, dead leaves, small shredded wood chips, dead pine needles, or compost. This is referred to as "mulching." Mulching your garden can reduce water loss and moderate temperature swings. During the hottest months, soil should remain covered if possible, as the sun can dry out and degrade the health of the soil. The only exception to this rule is during very wet months or early spring, when slugs and snails thrive in heavily mulched areas of the garden. Scraping back mulch in early spring can temporarily help to warm the soil and encourage seed germination.

Dealing with Pests

There is good news about pests and medicinal herbs: Most herbs either repel pests or attract beneficial insects that help keep pest populations in check. So the more herbs you grow, the more you will attract pollinators and "good" bugs that like to eat the more destructive pests, which will lead to a more successful garden!

When it comes to managing pests in the garden, it's important to remember that you are altering the ecosystem of an area that existed on its own before you planted anything into it. So the first couple years in a new garden can feel like wave after wave of pests are overtaking your plants. This is normal. The goal of a long-term healthy garden is to work *with* the environment you are trying to cultivate to allow the plants, pollinators, and even the annoying pests to balance out. Immediately attempting to remove a new pest entirely from your garden will only further these initial imbalances and prolong the process of helping your garden grow better on its own. Still, you may periodically find some destructive bugs on your herbs, so it's good to know what to do when that happens without taking an overly aggressive approach.

APHIDS

Aphids are tiny, sap-sucking insects that cluster on stems and leaf undersides, especially on stressed plants. Stressed plants have lowered defense mechanisms, and therefore can attract these types of pests. If you see aphids, don't panic. Think of them as a signal that your plants need some attention.

Treating Aphids

First, spray the aphids off with a steady stream of water daily to reduce the population and minimize the damage they may be causing to the plant. Then assess the other factors that may be causing the core issue for that plant:

- Is it experiencing watering consistency and/or drainage issues?
- Does this herb have poor airflow among its stems or branches?
- Is the herb located in sun/heat that is too harsh in the afternoons?
- Is this herb growing in soil that's too cold?

Sometimes addressing these issues can help your plants overcome an aphid infestation. But other times you may not catch this infestation early enough, and that's when ladybugs can save the day.

Ladybugs are ferocious aphid eaters, and when they have a food source and a few host plants to lay their eggs on and use for shelter while they hunt smaller pests, you may find that they show up with very little effort on your part. Ladybugs' favorite plants to host on are dill, fennel, cilantro, alyssum, chives, calendula, and yarrow. So if you want to invite ladybugs into your garden, plant these herbs! (Note: Purchasing live ladybugs is generally discouraged. Most won't remain in your garden unless the habitat suits them, and it can be environmentally harmful to add them, since many are harvested from nonlocal populations, raising ethical concerns about introducing non-native species to your garden.)

Alternatively, you can spray the leaves of your plants with a store-bought seaweed emulsion or worm casting tea. This is called a "foliar spray" because the treatment is sprayed directly on the foliage (the leaves) of your plants. Such amendments can help reduce your plants' stress level and boost their ability to fight off large-scale pest infestations.

Sometimes young plants don't survive an aphid infestation, and that's okay. There's no need to use harsh pesticides or attempt to remove all aphids if you have them in your garden. If some aphids stick around, it's not a failure on your part but a necessary step in the process of helping build a more balanced ecosystem for future seasons, because now the ladybugs know where the aphid buffet is.

SPIDER MITES

Spider mites are technically not spiders (though they resemble them up close) but are very tiny mites that you can barely see moving. They look like tiny little black or red dots on the underside of leaves, and they suck out the sap and energy from the plant's leaves.

It's best to try to notice spider mites as quickly as possible to avoid plant damage. You can periodically check the undersides of your plant's leaves to see if there are mites present. The first sign of actual damage is the leaves of your plant turning a silvery or whiter hue. When you examine the leaves closely, it can look like tons of tiny individual white spots on them. Spider mites will create a telltale web on the plant's leaves in the later stages of infestation that makes them easy to identify at that point. Spider mites thrive in hot, dry conditions and reproduce rapidly.

Herbs that spider mites tend to take hold of are the same herbs that prefer similar conditions. So woody-stemmed herbs, like lavender and rosemary, can be a target for spider mite infestations, especially midsummer. Spider mites can also take over indoor plants quickly, so keep an eye out and utilize all treatments at the first sign of damage.

Treating Spider Mites

Treatment for spider mites can be tricky. Since these pests love hot, dry conditions, misting your plants daily for a few weeks can help slow the spread and create less favorable conditions for this pest to thrive.

If spider mites persist, you can make a homemade bee-safe treatment:

- ¼ teaspoon peppermint essential oil
- ¼ teaspoon rosemary essential oil
- 1 tablespoon castile soap
- 1 quart water
- 1 teaspoon olive oil

Combine thoroughly and spray on plants daily in the evening for 2 weeks to manage spider mite populations.

You can also spray the leaves of your plants with a store-bought seaweed emulsion or worm casting tea. Just like with aphid infestations, plants that are stressed can become magnets for spider mites as well, so addressing plant stress is the best way to stop recurring infestations.

FUNGUS GNATS

Indoor herbs are more prone to fungus gnats, which lay larvae in wet soil and damage roots. Without exposure to outdoor elements, containers can hold on to too much moisture. A very moist environment can create the perfect breeding ground for this pest. Some store-bought potting mixes can even come with fungus gnat larvae already present in the bags.

Treating Fungus Gnats

Address the larval stage of the fungus gnat by mixing 1 part hydrogen peroxide with 8 parts water, then use it to drench the soil of your plants every 4–6 days. Address the adult fungus gnat by placing yellow sticky traps in or near your plants

for indoor infestations. Avoid using yellow sticky traps for outdoor treatments as beneficial pollinators can get stuck in them.

Diseases and Treatments

Fungal diseases, like rust, leaf spot, and powdery mildew, can affect herbs in your garden. Poor airflow can increase the risk of these issues developing, so stay on top of pruning to increase airflow inside the plant's structure.

RUST

Rust is a disease that looks very similar to actual rust, with orange, yellow, or brown spores on the underside of the leaves. Leaves may turn yellow or brown and prematurely drop from the plant.

Treating Rust

Treatment includes removal of diseased plant parts, pruning to improve airflow, and potentially using a sulfur-based fungicide if large parts of the garden are affected. Avoiding overhead watering can help stop this problem from happening in the first place. Instead, water near the base of the plant.

LEAF SPOTS

Leaf spots show up as brown or black spots, often with a yellow halo. They are spread through splashing water or shared tools.

Treating Leaf Spots

Be sure to sterilize shears, pruners, and other tools in between caring for different plants to avoid spreading this fungus. Avoid watering overhead and consider treating with an organic fungicide to knock back the infection.

POWDERY MILDEW

Powdery mildew is more common during transitional months with warm days and cooler nights, and it looks like white powder on the leaves. It typically affects herbs like basil, oregano, mint, and lemon balm.

Treating Powdery Mildew

To treat powdery mildew, first remove any affected leaves. If all leaves are affected, remove just the worst-looking leaves. Treat by spraying the affected leaves with any one of these three DIY solutions daily:

- 1 part cow's milk to 8 parts water
- 1 part baking soda to 8 parts water
- 1 part hydrogen peroxide to 8 parts water

ROOT ROT AND FUSARIUM WILT

Root rot and fusarium wilt are two soil-borne illnesses that show similar symptoms: sudden wilting and rotting stems with a foul smell. These two diseases can be confused for one another as they present similarly. They primarily affect herbaceous, tender-stemmed herbs, but can affect woody-stemmed herbs as well.

Treating Root Rot and Fusarium Wilt

To avoid root rot and fusarium wilt in the first place, practice proper pruning and plant spacing for optimal airflow to reduce trapped moisture, sterilize your equipment, and avoid overhead watering by only watering at the base of the plants. To sterilize your tools, wipe or spray the parts of the tools that have contact with plants and soil with 70% rubbing alcohol and let dry.

- **Root rot:** If you already have signs of root rot, you can attempt to remove the affected plants and repot them into drier soil mixes while using a lighter watering schedule to help them dry out. A mixture of 1 part hydrogen peroxide to 8 parts water can be poured into the soil to help kill off fungal diseases as well.
- **Fusarium wilt:** If you believe you have true fusarium wilt in your garden, remove the affected plants and throw them away. (Do not add them to your compost, as this type of disease can be spread via the soil throughout the garden.) Consider solarizing the infected areas of your garden by covering moist soil with clear or black plastic for 4–6 weeks to kill pathogens with heat in the hottest months. Try growing resistant varieties of herbs, like Nufar basil, if this fungus persists in your garden.

Proper Pruning and Harvesting Techniques

Regular pruning helps herbs grow fuller, stay healthy, and produce more leaves and flowers. Whether you are pruning to harvest (trimming the plant with the purpose of using the cuttings) or to maintain shape (trimming pieces from the plant as a form of maintenance, whether you utilize those cuttings or not), timing matters. Here are some general guidelines:

- Try to keep your pruners sharpened and clean between uses. To sterilize your tools, wipe or spray the parts of the tools that have contact with plants and soil with 70% rubbing alcohol and let dry.
- A light trim during the growing season encourages branching, which leads to bushier plants and more harvestable material.
- For the highest medicinal potency in herbs, harvest in the mornings.
- For heavy summer pruning, trim in the evening so plants can recover overnight.

Don't stress if you can't always follow these rules; your plants will still survive! The following information is about how to prune specific types of herbs.

WOODY HERBS

Pruning woody herbs can promote healthy airflow within the plant and encourage healthy new growth. But timing is important. For example, there is an 8-8 rule for lavender in zones 5–8 in the South. Prune lavender by August 8, leaving at least 8" of green growth on the plant to harden off before winter. For most woody-stemmed herbs, you can safely perform major shaping and pruning after the plant is done flowering, but 6–8 weeks before your first frost of the season is expected. This gives any new growth a bit of time to harden before winter cold arrives.

Avoid pruning woody-stemmed herbs back to the woody base. They don't regenerate from old brown wood stems. Leaving some soft green growth can give the plant a platform to continue its growth.

HERBACEOUS (TENDER-STEMMED) HERBS

Pruning tender herbs, like basil and lemon balm, keeps them bushy and prevents bolting. If your herbs tend to grow tall and floppy, pruning them at the leaf nodes about halfway up the stem can help them send out more branches from those points. This gives a bushier appearance to most tender herbs when done regularly. Bolting is the natural flowering and seeding process that often changes the herb's flavor to a less desirable one.

The life cycle for annuals involves the plant being started from seed, growing to a certain stage, and eventually being triggered to "reproduce" by forming flowers, which then dry and create seeds that would naturally fall to the ground or be carried by the wind and animals to other areas (bolting).

Even with regular pruning, annual plants will eventually bolt. Once this officially starts, their flavor will inevitably change. You can slow this process by pruning the plant regularly, which tells the plant it needs to keep producing more leaves or stems instead of flowers and seeds.

How to Propagate Herbs

Many herbs can be propagated, or reproduced, from cuttings or root divisions, creating entirely new plants.

PROPAGATING HERBACEOUS HERBS

Save some healthy cuttings after pruning. For soft-stemmed herbs, like basil or mint, place the cutting in a sunny windowsill with just the base of the stem touching water. Change the water every few days. Roots should start to appear within a week or two.

PROPAGATING WOODY HERBS

Woody herbs may take longer to form roots and can rot in water, so you want to use a different technique to propagate these types of herbs. Dip the end of the woody cutting into a rooting hormone and then plant it in a well-draining potting mix. There are a few different options for rooting hormones, such as commercially made ones or homemade options like cinnamon, honey, or aloe vera. Make sure to keep the potting mix consistently moist for 2–3 weeks until roots form.

DIVIDING PERENNIAL HERBS VIA ROOTS

Some perennial herbs can be divided at the roots to create new plants. This process is called "root division propagation." There are two main ways to do this: crown divisions and root cuttings.

Plants like comfrey or valerian grow deep taproots but eventually form a root "crown," with smaller new crowns that form new plants. For this type of root propagation, you can take pieces of the root crown that look like mini crowns themselves and replant them to create new plants. To choose a viable section of the root crown, look for a cluster of at least three to five root stems connected to top growth (the leaves) of the plants.

To take root cuttings, cut off pieces of the root that are 2–6" long and about the diameter of a pencil or thicker, replant them either in small pots or in another spot in the ground, and monitor them for new growth. Keep any divisions or cuttings consistently moist in the first few weeks of growth.

Plants that are aggressive spreaders, like mint and lemon balm, can be divided by their rhizomatous (root system) underground growth. To snag a new section, you can dig up just one portion of the plant that contains both roots and aboveground growth and plop it into a new pot! This chunk of your original plant will eventually grow into its own once it's given water and soil space to spread out its own roots.

Designing an Herb Garden

Now that you understand the different types of herbs and how they grow, you can begin to think about what your garden or growing area will look like. This section will walk you through the many factors to consider when planning your herb garden.

WHAT ARE YOUR GOALS?

Before you start designing your space, it's important to first decide on your garden's purpose. Do you want to maintain a steady supply of herbal teas? Cultivate specific herbs to address your health needs? Or grow a variety of things to have a range of herbal remedies at the ready? Or maybe you want to create a beautiful space to enjoy that *also* provides medicinal benefits.

Next, consider the logistical questions. Do you have lots of space to work with, or are you using a few containers for growing? Do you need to consider homeowners' association rules? Realistically, how much time do you see yourself having available to maintain your space on a daily and weekly basis?

Finally, when designing any garden, it's important to also support and enrich your local environment. For example, you can actively support pollinators by planting diverse host plants and food sources with the goal of creating a balance between what both you and nature need to live in harmony.

Now that you've considered your goals, you can move on to some of the logistical questions for your garden.

CHOOSING THE RIGHT LOCATION: SUNNY AND SHADY SPOTS

Most herbs thrive in sunny, well-drained spots with 6–8 hours of sunlight per day. If you're not sure which areas get sun, start to observe potential spots on a sunny day to track the light.

Outdoors

Outdoors, choose a spot that gets morning sun, has good airflow, and allows for easy watering and harvesting. Here are some additional tips for considering light in outdoor gardens:

- Woody perennials tolerate intense sun and drier conditions, while soft-stemmed herbs prefer more moisture and may benefit from afternoon shade, specifically in hotter climates.
- If you are container gardening in hot climates, your containers should be large (5 gallons or larger) to protect root health and moisture levels.
- Shade-loving herbs, like lemon balm, mint, and skullcap, can be tucked into the cooler corners of your garden in partial shade.
- Woody herbs should be placed in the higher areas of your garden in full sun with good drainage. If you can't control the ground drainage, consider planting woody herbs in large containers instead.

Indoors

If you're growing indoors or on a balcony, a south-facing window or bright patio will work best. Most herbs do best with 6–8 hours of sunlight a day. If sunlight is limited, a grow light can help leafy herbs thrive. There are a lot of great and affordable options available nowadays when it comes to grow lights. LED options reduce ambient heat and energy usage. (A windowsill is a great space for starting seeds or propagating cuttings, but many medicinal herbs may outgrow it.)

Container Growing

Growing herbs in containers offers flexibility, especially in small spaces, like patios or balconies. Containers allow you to move plants with the seasons, optimize sun exposure, and control aggressive spreaders, like mint. They also allow you to control drainage. Here are some tips for growing certain types of herbs in containers:

- **Woody-stemmed herbs,** like rosemary or lavender, need pots that are 12–18" wide and 18–24" deep at a minimum to develop strong root systems that can withstand temperature swings. Use containers with multiple drainage holes and consider placing them on sliders or dollies if they are large to help with moving tender plants that need winter protection.
- **For herbaceous/tender herbs,** you have more wiggle room on container sizes. For example, basil can grow well in a pot sized anywhere from 4" to 1 gallon on a sunny windowsill or patio. If you use a smaller container, be sure to

maintain a regular watering schedule, because tender herbs dry out faster, especially in summer months.

- **For spreading herbs,** like mint, containers are a great solution, but there are some best practices when going for this option. Use saucers under your mint pots to avoid the root systems invading nearby soil through drainage holes. Mint also loves bottom watering and shady spots, so placing your container in a saucer in the shade creates ideal conditions.
- **Taproot herbs** often struggle in containers because they can't reach deep for water and nutrients. While regular fertilization can help, these plants generally do better in the ground or in raised beds with open bottoms.

Raised Bed or In-Ground Growing

Most medicinal and culinary herbs thrive in raised or in-ground garden beds, but choosing the best option depends on your local soil conditions. Some areas of the southern United States have clay soil that is rich in minerals but often drains poorly. Coastal areas, like Florida, tend to have more sandy soil that drains very well but struggles to hold on to nutrients. Both types of soil can benefit from seasonal additions of compost, which loosens clay and helps sand retain moisture.

If your native soil contains limestone, contaminants, or other issues that make in-ground growing difficult, raised beds can offer a safe and more controlled alternative. There are a range of depths when it comes to raised bed options, but most herbs can benefit from even 6" of decent quality soil for putting down roots.

LET YOUR HERBS WORK TOGETHER

When planning your herb list, group plants by growth habit to help them support one another. You can even start with one herb in the center of your space, then plan around it based on plant needs and habits. For example, ground cover herbs (low-growing, spreading herbs that cover the soil as they grow), like self-heal, act as living mulch by reducing evaporation, protecting soil health, and helping regulate root temperature. Taller herbs, like basil, can offer beneficial shade to these lower growers.

You can also help protect your plant's roots and soil health by adding wood chips, straw, or dead leaves to any open areas of soil.

Herbs with deep taproots, like Russian Bocking 14 comfrey, help break up compacted soil and draw nutrients from deep below the surface. These plants thrive as understory companions, which get this distinction because they grow underneath the shade of larger plants, like trees. They can tolerate a more humid environment and help protect the soil for the larger plants—they work together in a mutually beneficial relationship. For example, comfrey doesn't like intense heat, so planting it beneath taller species creates a small protective microclimate.

BOOSTING VISUAL APPEAL WITH FLOWERING HERBS

As you design your garden, don't forget about color. Herbs often bloom, which can help balance out the look of a medicinal herb garden in a typical landscape. Flowering plants in general typically need the most sun to help them have enough energy to produce those blooms, so opt for a sunnier location for herbs in this category. Here are some herbs that can add color to your space:

- **Lavender:** Spikes of purple blooms with a strong perfume.
- **Chamomile:** Small, daisy-like flowers with a sweet, apple-like aroma.
- **Calendula:** Bright orange or yellow blooms with sticky petals and medicinal resin.
- **Echinacea:** Upright clusters of medium pink coneflowers that spread to a larger patch each year. (Other colors of this flower do exist—ask your local garden center for some ideas.)

SHOULD YOU START FROM SEED OR SEEDLINGS?

Annual herbs, like basil, chamomile, and cilantro, grow quickly from seed. Some seeds are simple to germinate as long as you follow the general rule of planting the seed at about the same depth as the size of the seed itself. But perennial woody herbs grow much slower from seed and tend to be more efficient to grow from propagations and live young plants that you can purchase from a nursery.

Starting plants from seed can save money, but if you are new to gardening it's best to start out with a mix of live plants and some beginner-friendly herb seeds to learn how the process works. In fact, seed starting your own plants is an entire skill set to learn on its own, and it can initially be frustrating. It may seem like you are working backward by growing live plants first, then moving onto starting from seed, but using seedlings allows you to start your garden in a much faster and easier way. Plus, it allows you to learn through observation of how the plants grow.

Understanding Cold Stratification

Some seeds need cold stratification to improve germination rates. Cold strati- fication is the process of exposing seeds to a period of cold, moist conditions that mimic the winter weather for seeds that would naturally resow themselves in the wild. This can be done by placing seeds in a damp paper towel in the fridge for 4–6 weeks before planting.

PLANT SPACING

One of the most common mistakes new gardeners make is not giving herbs enough space to reach their full size. For example, herbs like rosemary can get *very* big and still need ample airflow to avoid disease. Consider planting rose- mary on its own with room for it to grow to a final size of 3–4'! Since rosemary is a slower-growing perennial, you can plant yearly annuals around it to fill in the empty space until it needs more breathing room,

if you don't like the emptiness that proper spacing can create for c few months.

Of course, space is also a consideration when planting in containers. Remember that herbs grown in containers may stay smaller due to limited root space. What thrives in a large garden bed might grow much more modestly in a pot, so plan your space accordingly.

Get Growing

This chapter gave you a very broad overview of the many factors that go into cultivating a medicinal herb garden. The best way to learn is by trying, so choose some plants and begin! The next chapter will show you how to use what you harvest to improve your well-be ng with various tinctures and salves.

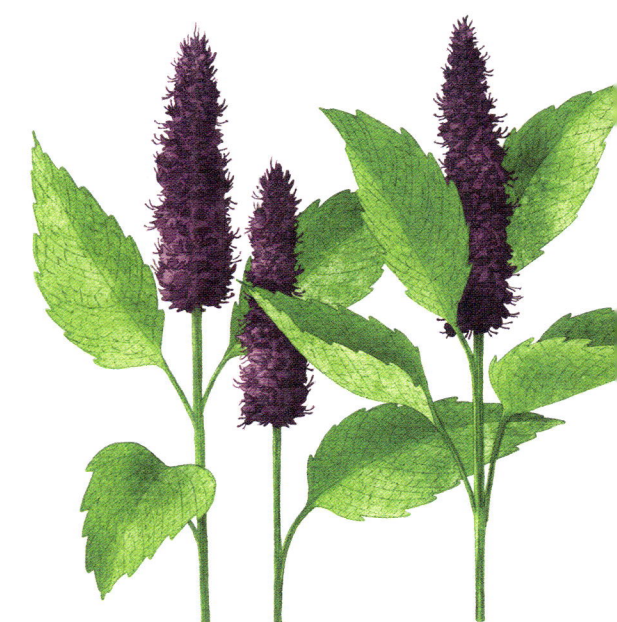

CHAPTER 2

Making Tinctures and Salves

The true magic of herbalism begins when you start working with your thriving plants to create healing options for yourself and others. Before you know it, you'll be able to take fresh or dried herbs from the garden or shelf and turn them into something useful.

In this chapter, we'll walk through the essentials of making tinctures, salves, poultices, and more. You'll learn about the tools you'll need, how to preserve herbs, and how different preparations support the body in unique ways. Two of the most useful and versatile preparations are tinctures (for internal use) and salves (for topical support). These simple methods extract and preserve a plant's beneficial properties and offer specific healing properties. By understanding the options within each category, you'll build a solid foundation for your herbal practice.

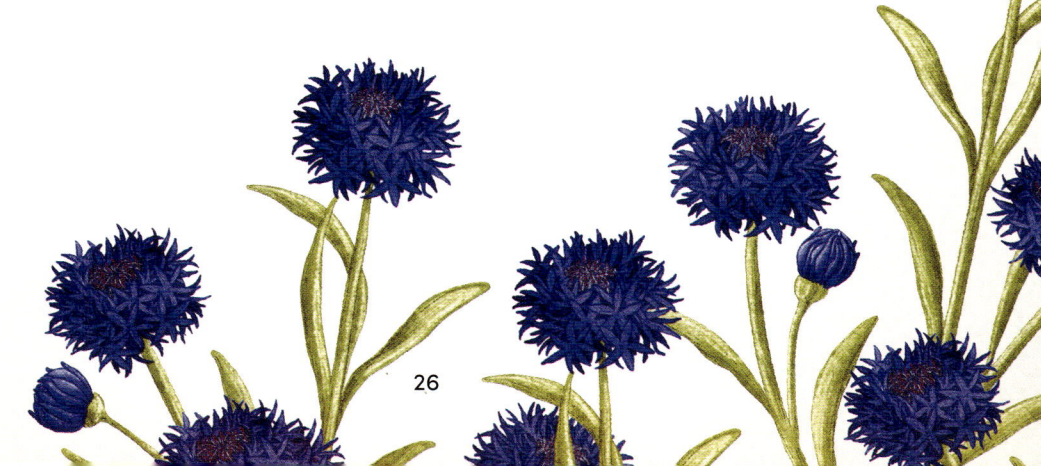

Understanding Herbal Properties

Each herb in this book has special qualities that can help you improve or maintain your health. The way that medicinal herbs work with our bodies can be classified into four main categories, known as the "energetics" of the herbs. These are either warming or cooling and drying or moistening. Getting to know which herbs have which properties helps you match the plant to what your body needs. For example:

- **Cooling** herbs, like peppermint and violet, calm heat, inflammation, or irritation in the body.
- **Warming** herbs, like ginger, are great for sluggish digestion and poor circulation.
- **Drying** herbs, like yarrow, may be helpful in treating damp conditions, like congestion, weepy skin issues, or excess mucus.
- **Moistening** herbs, like marshmallow root and licorice, soothe dryness in the throat, skin, and digestive system.

By learning to recognize your body's needs, you can choose herbs to restore harmony instead of just chasing symptoms.

HERBAL CONTRAINDICATIONS

Another good reason to learn herbal properties is so that you don't accidentally make a condition worse. Even gentle herbs can cause issues if they're not a good fit for what your body needs. For example:

- Warming herbs may worsen hot flashes and night sweats.
- Drying herbs can aggravate dry skin, chronic dehydration, or dry coughs.
- Moistening herbs may not be helpful for excess mucus, candida, or bloat.

Plus, it's always important to talk to your doctor about what you're using because some herbs interact with medications, affect blood pressure, or influence hormones.

Choosing Extraction Methods

When it comes to actually extracting the beneficial properties from your medicinal herbs, it's important to understand what an herbal constituent is and what type of solvent will best extract each type of constituent from each herb.

An herbal constituent is a naturally occurring chemical compound in a plant that contributes to its flavor, aroma, and medicinal action. The majority of the compounds we aim to extract into medicinal products are considered "organic constituents," which means they are made by the plant. There are also inorganic constituents, like minerals, that are absorbed from the soil, then concentrated in leaves, roots, and flowers.

Here are some examples of organic constituents:

- **Volatile essential oils:** Aromatic compounds that can affect the nervous system.

- **Alkaloids:** Potent nitrogen-based plant chemicals that often taste bitter and strongly affect the body.
- **Tannins:** Astringent plant compounds that dry and tone tissues.
- **Mucilage:** A soothing, protective "plant gel" that eases irritation and dryness.

In the context of herbal extractions, a solvent is the liquid used to dissolve and extract the active constituents from plant material. Different solvents pull out different types of compounds (constituents), so the choice of solvent determines what properties the finished remedy will have. Here are some common solvents in herbal medicine:

- **Water:** Extracts minerals, mucilage, and some alkaloids.
- **Alcohol:** Extracts alkaloids, polyphenols, flavonoids, sesquiterpene lactones, glycosides, resins, tannins, volatile essential oils, and some mucilage.
- **Glycerin:** Extracts glycosides, polyphenols, flavonoids, some tannins, and mucilage.
- **Vinegar:** Extracts minerals, alkaloids, glycosides, some polyphenols, and flavonoids.
- **Oil:** Extracts volatile essential oils, resins, and fat-soluble compounds.

Once you know the best solvent for extracting the medicinal properties of the herb you're planning to work with, you can move on to gathering the supplies needed to make your final product.

Tools of the Trade

When it comes to processing herbs after harvest and extracting compounds from your medicinal herbs, there are no strict requirements for tools you need to get the job done. But gathering some of these supplies can make the task a lot easier.

The following tools are great to have on hand for harvesting, preparing, and transforming herbs into salves, tinctures, and other remedies. You don't need everything at once, so just start with what you're most likely to need right away and build as you go.

FOR HARVESTING AND DRYING

- **Sharp garden snips or scissors:** For clean, precise cuts when harvesting herbs without damaging the plant.
- **Harvest baskets or mesh bags:** To help keep herbs from wilting or sweating before you process them.
- **Dehydrator with temperature control:** For drying delicate herbs quickly without losing their medicinal qualities.
- **Twine and herb drying racks:** For hanging bundles or laying herbs out to air-dry in a shaded, breezy spot.
- **Paper bags with ventilation holes:** For catching seeds or petals during drying while keeping dust and light out.

FOR TINCTURES AND GLYCERITES

- **Glass jars with tight-fitting lids:** Mason jars work well for infusing herbs in alcohol or glycerin. Clear glass is fine for infusing, but you'll want to store finished tinctures in amber or cobalt bottles to protect them from light.

- **High-proof alcohol (like vodka or Everclear):** Used as a solvent to extract medicinal compounds. Glycerin can be used for nonalcoholic alternatives.
- **Labels and a permanent marker:** Always date and label your jars with the herb name, medium (alcohol, glycerin, etc.), and ratio. A label maker or waterproof labels can help keep everything legible, even when exposed to oils or humidity.
- **Strainers, cheesecloth, or muslin:** For separating the plant material after infusing. Nut milk bags are great reusable options for filtering fine particulates. They are sturdy enough to squeeze without tearing, and you can easily wash them.
- **Funnel and dropper bottles:** For bottling up your finished tinctures in a clean, spill-free way that is easy for dosing.

FOR SALVES AND INFUSED OILS

- **Double boiler or a makeshift version (glass bowl over a pot):** For gently heating herbs in oil or melting waxes and butter without overheating.
- **Canning funnel:** A wide-mouthed funnel that fits Mason jars and can help reduce mess when transferring infused oils.
- **Small fine-mesh strainer:** Useful when combined with the canning funnel to quickly strain smaller amounts of plant material out of infused oils into a clean jar.

- **Carrier oil (like olive, jojoba, or coconut):** Used to extract and carry herbal properties into your skin
- **Beeswax or plant-based wax:** A key ingredient for thickening oils into salves and balms.
- **Small tins or glass jars:** To pour your finished salves into. Make sure they're sterilized and dry.
- **Wooden spoon or silicon spatula:** A tool dedicated to herbal use for stirring your oils and salves.
- **Mini whisk or electric mixer:** For blending salves, creams, or body butters into a smooth, even consistency.

POULTICES AND COMPRESSES

- **Mortar and pestle or food processor:** To mash or blend fresh herbs into a paste for poultices.
- **Gauze or muslin squares:** To wrap up poultices or herbal material for compresses.
- **Small saucepan or kettle:** For heating water to soak compress cloths or prepare herbal infusions.

PREPARATION AND MEASURING

- **Digital kitchen scale:** For measuring herbs and ingredients by weight, which can deliver more exact measurements and ratios calculations.
- **Small notebook or herbal journal:** To keep track of your recipes, ratios, harvest notes, and outcomes.
- **Measuring cups:** For following recipes or scaling up batches.

- **Thermometer:** For ensuring oils don't overheat and for monitoring temperatures when working with beeswax, glycerin, or butters.
- **PH test strips:** Helpful when formulating skincare items like toners or scrubs to ensure skin-safe acidity.

TEAS AND DECOCTIONS

- **French press or tea infuser:** For making loose-leaf tea infusions and decoctions without straining through a cloth each time.
- **Timer or phone alarm:** To measure how long your herbs have been steeping. Timing matters more than you'd think, especially with stronger infusions.
- **Kettle with temperature settings:** Herbal teas are most effective when consumed on a regular basis, so make it easy to prepare a cup of tea. Electric kettles can brew quickly and allow temperature control to maximize potency of herbs.

SPECIALTY EQUIPMENT

- **Slow cooker:** For making infused oils over low heat for several hours without having to babysit the stove.
- **Immersion blender:** Useful for emulsifications.
- **Coffee or herb grinder:** For grinding dried roots, barks, or leaves into powder for teas or capsules.
- **Capsule machine and empty capsules:** If you're making your own herbal supplements.

Different Ways to Dehydrate Herbs

When you're first starting to dehydrate herbs, you can often use tools you already have on hand. Regardless of the specific way you choose to hang your herbs to dry, you'll want to aim for a well-ventilated area with lower humidity and indirect light.

Let's dive into the pros and cons of the many dehydration options that are available to use.

Paper Sacks

One simple method is placing freshly cut herbs into paper lunch sacks with a few holes punched in the upper portion for airflow. To hang sacks (which ensures proper airflow), string a line between two nails and use clothespins to hang the bags.

Pros:
- Helps keep dust off the herbs and catches any petals or seeds that may fall during drying.
- You can easily label each bag with the date of harvest and name of the herb.

Cons:
- This method is not as efficient for processing larger volumes of herbs.
- If you are also concerned with the aesthetics of hang drying herbs, this method can be a bit unsightly.

Herb Bundles

You've probably seen bundles of herbs tied on strings across windowsills. While beautiful, this method comes with considerations.

Pros:
- Aesthetically appealing.
- Great for small batches of dried herbs that you're using in regular rotation.

Cons:
- High humidity can lead to mold on herbs that dry too slowly.
- A south-facing window may expose them to too much direct sunlight, which can degrade color and potency.
- You may end up with a mess of dropped leaves or seeds.
- Herbs hung over a sink can increase moisture during drying and cause mold.

Herb-Drying Racks

You can make your own herb-drying racks using mesh or screen material attached to old picture frames, in place of glass. Then, simply spread herbs out over the screens in a single layer and lay the frames flat in a well-ventilated area to allow herbs to dry gently but efficiently. You can also find store-bought herb-drying baskets, which often have zipped enclosures and layers and hang easily, keeping herbs contained and well ventilated.

Pros:
- Best for large amounts of herb drying at a time.
- Good for drying at gentle temperatures, which can preserve the delicate properties in some herbs.

Cons:
- Can potentially be a risk for mold developing if the environment you air-dry in is too humid or lacks airflow.
- Some herbs lose color if temps are too low and the dehydration process draws out, or if temps are too high.
- May require some DIY knowledge or resourcefulness, or a purchase of a product.

Electric Dehydrator

If you live in a very humid climate or have large amounts of herbs to harvest regularly, it may be worth investing in an electric dehydrator. Choose one with a temperature control that goes as low as 90–95°F to preserve the medicinal properties of delicate herbs.

Pros:
- A dehydrator will dry herbs faster and often preserve their color and flavor better than air-drying.

Cons:
- Electric dehydrators—especially ones that are a decent size and have specific temperature settings—can be expensive.

Basics of Making a Tincture

WHAT IS A TINCTURE?

A tincture is a concentrated liquid herbal extract made by soaking plant material in a solvent, most often alcohol, to dissolve and preserve the plant's active constituents. This process draws out the active compounds from the plant, preserving them for long-term use. Tinctures are usually taken in small doses by mouth, either on or under the tongue. Sometimes they are diluted in water or juice to help make the strong flavor of the herbs or alcohol more palatable.

WHAT TYPES OF HERBS ARE BEST FOR TINCTURES?

Tinctures are ideal for herbs that contain constituents that dissolve well in alcohol. Here are some examples of herbs that work well in tinctures: echinacea, valerian root, elecampane root, licorice root, motherwort, St.-John's-wort, skullcap, yarrow, horehound, mugwort, anise hyssop, passion vine, and blue vervain.

FRESH VERSUS DRIED HERB TINCTURES

Some herbs have constituents that are delicate and may not survive the dehydration process, so fresh herbs are best for tinctures when you want to capture delicate aromatics, pigments, or resins that fade during drying. Dried herbs are best for sturdy roots, barks, and plants that maintain their properties better during the drying process. For example, mint, lemon balm, catnip, oregano, thyme, and rosemary benefit from fresh tincturing to preserve their aroma and potency (although you can still extract many of their benefits from dried herbal preparations). St.-John's-wort contains a specific constituent called hyperforin that degrades more quickly after harvest, which is why fresh herb tinctures are considered stronger and more effective for this herb.

Resinous herbs, like calendula, yield more of the sticky constituent into alcohol before they dry out, and some juicy or delicate herbs, like holy basil and motherwort, benefit more from fresh tincturing.

UNDERSTANDING ALCOHOL PERCENTAGES

Alcohol is not just used for extracting constituents in tinctures but also for preservation of the extract. When making tinctures with fresh herbs, it's important to consider the extra water amounts that fresh herbs contain. This water will end up in your final product, therefore diluting the alcohol. This is why it is suggested to use a higher-proof alcohol when tincturing fresh herbs, to maintain a total alcohol percentage above the preservation threshold for the final product (25–30% alcohol). Different herbs may also require different alcohol percentages to pull the constituents from them for medicinal usage, so it's key to learn how to dilute alcohol to a specific percentage.

Alcohol content in liquids you buy is measured by what's called "proof" in the United States, or percent alcohol by volume (ABV).

Proof = 2 × the percent ABV. (So 80 proof = 40% alcohol.)

If the alcohol you have is stronger than you need, you can dilute it with distilled water.

Tips for Tincturing with Alcohol

- Vodka is a 40% (80 proof) alcohol, which works fine for extracting constituents from most herbs.
- Use higher-proof alcohol, like Everclear (95% ABV/190 proof), only when an herb is resinous or fresh, or when you know it needs more strength to extract a compound.
- You can always dilute strong alcohol with water, but you can't make weak alcohol stronger.
- Always use distilled water when diluting alcohol to avoid contaminants being added to your tincture. This can reduce chances of spoilage.

Here are some basic alcohol dilution calculations:

- Equal parts alcohol + water = alcohol strength cut to about half (~50%).
- 1 part alcohol + 2 parts water = alcohol strength cut to about a third (~30%).
- 2 parts alcohol + 1 part water = alcohol strength cut to about two-thirds (~60%).

Let's walk through some examples.

Example 1: You have 95% (190 proof) alcohol and want 50% alcohol.
50 divided by 95 = 0.53.

That 0.53 tells you that you want to keep about half of the alcohol. To do this, mix 1 cup 95% alcohol + 1 cup water, and you'll get a final product that's about 50% alcohol.

Example 2: You have 95% alcohol and want 30% alcohol.
30 divided by 95 = 0.32.

The 0.32 tells you that you want to keep about one-third of the alcohol. To do this, mix 1 cup 95% alcohol + 2 cups water, and you'll get a final product that's about 30% alcohol.

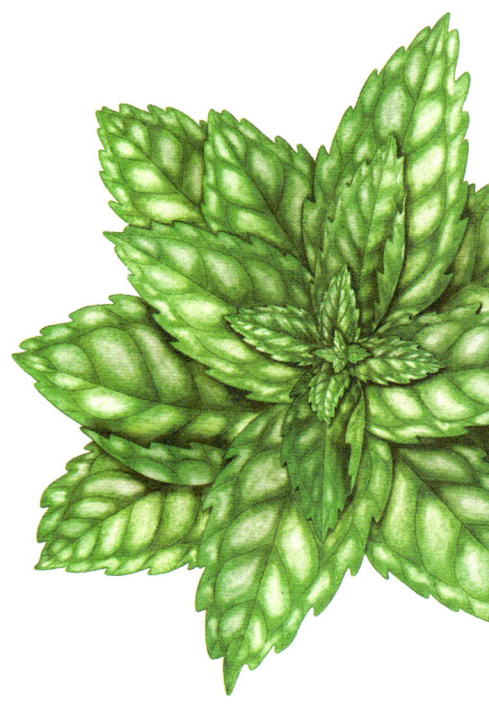

Basic Fresh Herb Tincture Recipe

WHAT YOU'LL NEED:

Clean glass jar with lid

Fresh herbs (chopped or crushed)

Specific alcohol percentage solution based on your chosen herb's constituents

Labels and permanent marker

Cheesecloth or fine-mesh strainer

Amber dropper bottle(s), for storage

WHAT TO DO:

1. Roughly chop your fresh herbs, pack them into a measuring cup to measure, and add them to a Mason jar.
2. Use a ratio of 1 part fresh herbs to 2 parts alcohol to calculate how much alcohol to add to your jar, making sure that your herbs are fully submerged under the volume of liquid in the jar.
3. Seal and label with the date and herb name.
4. Store in a cool, dark place for 4–6 weeks, shaking gently every few days.
5. After steeping, strain using cheesecloth or a fine-mesh strainer.
6. Transfer to amber dropper bottle(s) and label for daily use.

Note: For at-home herbalism, the measuring cup method gives a safe, reliable result. If you would like to be more precise with your measurements, you can utilize a scale to weigh herbs and measure liquids by grams or milliliters.

Basic Dried Herb Tincture Recipe

WHAT YOU'LL NEED:

Dried herbs

Clean glass jar with lid

Specific alcohol percentage solution based on your chosen herb's constituents

Labels and permanent marker

Cheesecloth or fine-mesh strainer

Amber dropper bottle(s), for storage

WHAT TO DO:

1. Roughly chop your dried herbs, pack them into a measuring cup to measure, and add them to a Mason jar.
2. Use a ratio of 1 part dried herbs to 5 parts alcohol to calculate how much alcohol to add to your jar, making sure that your herbs are fully submerged under the volume of liquid in the jar.
3. Seal and label with the date and herb name.
4. Store in a cool, dark place for 4–6 weeks, shaking gently every few days.
5. After steeping, strain using cheesecloth or a fine-mesh strainer.
6. Transfer to amber dropper bottle(s) and label for daily use.

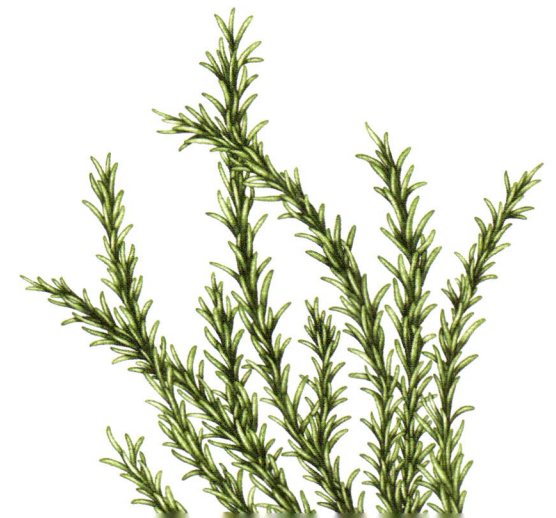

GLYCERITES AND TINCTURE ALTERNATIVES

Glycerites are alcohol-free herbal extracts made using food-grade vegetable glycerin. They're sweet, shelf-stable for about a year, and ideal for children or anyone avoiding alcohol. While glycerin isn't as strong of a solvent as alcohol, it still does a great job extracting many medicinal properties. For example, it is very effective when used with soothing, moistening, or aromatic herbs, like lemon balm, anise hyssop, or chamomile. Use dried herbs when possible to prevent spoilage and store your finished glycerites in a cool, dark place.

You can also extract some medicinal properties from herbs using vinegar to make an acetum. Although this preparation may not be as potent in terms of medicinal use, it can be tasty and used in salad dressings or daily tonics. Honey-based infusions, called oxymels, can be a tasty alternative to tinctures as well. See more about these preparations in Chapter 3 of this book.

Salves

WHAT IS A SALVE?

A salve is a semisolid herbal preparation made by infusing herbs into oil and then thickening the oil with beeswax or a beeswax alternative. Salves are used externally on the skin to soothe and heal skin irritations. Similar skin-soothing herbal infusions can be made using other fats, like shea butter and tallow, for balms and body butters. Salves are very useful because:

- They can address dry, irritated, or damaged skin.
- You can customize them to manage specific skin issues.
- They're shelf-stable and easy to apply.

WHAT TYPES OF HERBS ARE BEST FOR SALVES?

Since salves start with an oil-based herbal infusion, opt for herbs that have fat-soluble constituents. Herbs that do well infused into salves include calendula, plantain, comfrey, rosemary, peppermint, lavender, and yarrow.

UNDERSTANDING CARRIER OILS

Carrier oils are natural products that help bring herbs safely to your skin. When choosing oils for salve making, it's helpful to consider their comedogenic rating. This is a scale from 0 to 5 that reflects how likely an oil is to clog pores. Oils with a lower rating, like jojoba, sunflower, or hemp seed oil, are less likely to cause breakouts and are generally better suited for facial salves or acne-prone skin. Richer oils, like coconut oil or cocoa butter, have higher comedogenic scores and may be better reserved for dry-skin salves or body balms.

Skin-Safe Oils	Number Rating	Explanation
Hempseed oil	0	Least likely to clog pores
Grape-seed oil	1	Very low likelihood of clogging pores
Jojoba oil	2	Low chance of clogging pores
Sweet almond oil	2	Low chance of clogging pores
Olive oil	3	Fairly high likelihood of clogging pores for some people
Coconut oil	4	Most likely to clog pores

Everyone's skin reacts differently, so it's worth experimenting with oils that suit your skin type, which can be even more important for products used on sensitive areas or for daily use.

UNDERSTANDING THICKENING AGENTS

Sometimes you want a product that's thicker than an oil, and that's where beeswax and other alternatives come in. To create a spreadable salve using your infused oils, you'll briefly melt the thickening agent and blend it with your warmed liquid herbal oil. As this mixture cools, it will thicken to a semisoft consistency. Beeswax is the most common thickening agent used in salves. It helps create a firm, stable texture while adding in a gentle protective barrier for the skin. It melts at around 145°F, and it should be gently heated using a double boiler to avoid scorching your infused oils. Beeswax comes in bricks and pellet forms. If you can source the pellets in pure beeswax form, they are ideal for easily measuring out in recipes.

Carnauba and candelilla wax are plant-based alternatives to beeswax. They have higher melting points, at 160–170°F, and they will create a firmer final product. So, you may need to adjust the ratio you use of this solid wax to the liquid oil in your recipe to reach your preferred consistency.

For example, if a recipe calls for 1 part beeswax, you can swap with $1/2$ part candelilla wax or $1/3$–$1/2$ part carnauba wax. Incorporating other skin-soothing fats, like shea butter or tallow, in addition to a carrier oil or thickening agent can enrich your salves, but it will also soften them, since fats like those can melt at cooler temperatures compared to beeswax.

HOW TO MAKE A BASIC SALVE

The base recipe for a salve is usually a ratio of 1 part (firm at room temperature) wax to 8 parts (liquid at room temperature) oil. For example, you might combine 1 tablespoon of wax to 8 tablespoons of oil or 1 ounce of wax by weight to 8 ounces of oil by weight. This ratio will give a medium firmness to your salve that should spread easily with the warmth of your hands.

You can increase the firm wax amount in this ratio to create what is considered a balm, or reduce the firm wax in this ratio to produce an ointment-like texture for the final product. Essentially, if you add anything to the base 1:8 recipe, it will impact the final product's texture. In fact,

you should avoid adding a higher ratio of softer fats, like tallow and shea butter, into your salves during the summer months if you live in a hotter climate to avoid them melting quickly inside your containers. In colder weather, however, those fat additions can be very soothing to dry skin, and cooler temperatures will help them stabilize their consistency during storage.

Also, keep in mind that waxes tend to coat utensils, pots, and jars, making them difficult to remove when cleaning. Rubbing alcohol is a great way to wipe down these tools to remove residue between uses, but eventually saving tools just for making salves can be helpful.

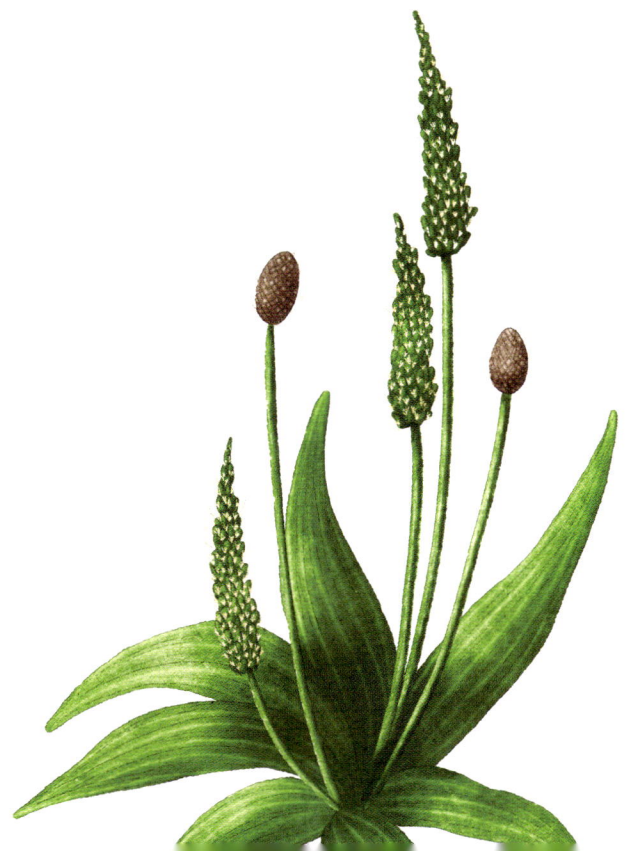

Basic Salve Recipe

WHAT YOU'LL NEED:

Clean glass jar with a lid

Dried herbs (like calendula, comfrey, or plantain)

A carrier oil

A double boiler (or a heat-safe bowl over a smaller pot of water)

Cheesecloth

Beeswax pellets

Tins or jars, for storage

Labels and permanent marker

WHAT TO DO:

1. To infuse the oil, fill a jar to the top with dried herbs and cover them completely in your skin-safe oil of choice. Seal and let the jar sit in a cool, dark place for 6 weeks (up to 6 months), or place the oil and herbs in a double boiler for 2 hours. You can also place the oil and herbs in a heat-safe, sealed glass jar inside of a slow cooker on low heat for 2–3 hours for a hands-off infusion. The key is to make sure the oil covers the herbs during this process. Using a water bath with a jar can help you avoid exposing your infusion to high temperatures for extended periods of time to avoid degrading the medicinal compounds of the herbs.

2. Strain the infused oil through a cheesecloth to remove the herbs. This is now a standalone herbal oil infusion.

3. In a double boiler over medium-high heat, combine 1 cup (8 ounces) of the infused oil with 1 ounce of beeswax.

4. Stir gently until the beeswax is fully melted. Beeswax can take a while to heat up enough to melt fully, so be patient.

5. Pour this mixture into tins or jars while it is still liquid and pourable, then let it cool slowly until firm. Seal and label for daily use.

Note: Some low-water flowering herbs like calendula, St.-John's-wort, chamomile, and lavender can be infused from a fresh state with a lower risk of spoilage. Simply harvest these herbs and let them wilt for a couple of hours before infusing into oil.

CONSIDERING PH LEVELS FOR WATER-BASED SKIN CARE

Products like salves and body butters don't contain water, so they don't affect skin pH or require preservatives. But if you're making lotions, toners, or soaps that include water, it's important to keep the pH between 4.5 and 5.5 to match the skin's natural barrier and prevent irritation or microbial growth.

To check the pH of your skin care, dip a pH test strip into a small sample of your finished product. Compare the color to the chart provided with the strips. Aim for a pH between 4.5–5.5. If the pH is too high (alkaline), a tiny amount of citric acid or diluted apple cider vinegar can help bring it back into range. You can use a dilution of 1 part apple cider vinegar to 9 parts distilled water and gradually add drops to your mixture, testing as you go. If the pH is too low (acidic), add very small amounts of baking soda (sodium bicarbonate) to increase the pH.

Cornflower and Rose Toner

This herbal facial toner soothes redness, hydrates, and reduces puffiness. The witch hazel is a cooling astringent, which can help reduce swelling and tone skin.

WHAT YOU'LL NEED:

1 cup distilled water

1 tablespoon dried cornflower petals

1 tablespoon dried rose petals

Cheesecloth

1 teaspoon witch hazel (alcohol-free; optional)

pH testing strips

Small spray bottle or toner bottle

WHAT TO DO:

1. In a small saucepan, bring water just to a boil and remove from heat.
2. Add dried petals, cover, and steep for 15–20 minutes.
3. Strain through a cheesecloth and cool completely. Add witch hazel at this stage if using.
4. Test pH and adjust if it falls under 4.5 or over 5.5.
5. Store in a spray or toner bottle in the fridge and use within 5–7 days.

Poultices and Compresses

WHAT ARE POULTICES AND COMPRESSES?

Herbal compresses and poultices are both used to apply herbs directly to the skin for localized healing. But they differ in how they're prepared.

HOW TO MAKE A BASIC POULTICE AND COMPRESS

- A **poultice** is made by mashing or grinding fresh or dried herbs into a paste and applying it directly to the skin. It's messy, but it delivers herbs in their raw, potent form. Poultices are great for drawing out infection, soothing bites, or easing inflammation.
- A **compress** is made by soaking a clean cloth in a strong herbal tea or infusion. After wringing the cloth out, it is laid over the affected area. Compresses are less messy than poultices and can be gentler for sore muscles, fevers, swollen joints, or irritated skin. They can also be used hot (for soothing cramps) or cold (to soothe overheated skin or swelling).

WHAT TYPES OF HERBS ARE BEST FOR POULTICES AND COMPRESSES?

These herbs work well in herbal compresses:

- **Lavender:** Antimicrobial and soothing, especially for cramps or headaches.
- **Plantain leaf:** For drawing out toxins and calming itches and bites.
- **Mint:** Cooling; helps with headaches, fevers, and sore muscles.
- **Chamomile:** Reduces swelling and soothes inflamed skin.
- **Yarrow:** Astringent; helpful for bruises, rashes, and broken capillaries.
- **Blue vervain:** Tension relief and cooling for neck or shoulder stress.
- **Sage:** Astringent; great for wound cleansing.
- **Thyme:** Antiseptic; helps with infections.

These herbs work well in herb poultices:

- **Comfrey:** Rich in allantoin; speeds cell repair; soothes bruises, sprains, and fractures.
- **Plantain leaf:** For drawing out toxins and calming itches and bites.
- **Yarrow:** Astringent; helpful for bruises, rashes, and broken capillaries; stops bleeding quickly.
- **Self-heal:** Speeds tissue repair and soothes minor wounds.
- **Calendula:** Promotes wound healing and tissue repair; soothes minor scrapes and burns.
- **Garlic:** Strong antimicrobial; used for boils and infections, but can irritate sensitive skin.
- **Rose petals:** Cooling; mildly astringent for inflamed skin.
- **Horehound:** Warming, drawing; used on the chest for cough and congestion.

Comfrey Poultice

Comfrey (*Symphytum officinale*) is a powerful herb traditionally used to support tissue repair, reduce inflammation, and help heal bruises, sprains, or minor injuries. A poultice allows you to apply comfrey's healing properties directly to the skin, where they're needed most.

WHAT YOU'LL NEED:

Fresh, or dried and rehydrated, comfrey leaves

Mortar and pestle, blender, or knife

Clean cloth, gauze, or muslin

WHAT TO DO:

1. Rinse fresh leaves and chop or crush them into a thick paste. If using dried, pour a bit of warm water over them until soft, then mash.
2. Apply the paste: Spread the mashed comfrey directly onto unbroken skin or onto a layer of cloth. If applying directly, cover with clean cloth to hold in place.
3. Secure and rest: Wrap cloth to hold poultice in place and leave for 20–40 minutes.
4. Remove and rinse the area. Repeat 1 or 2 times daily if needed.

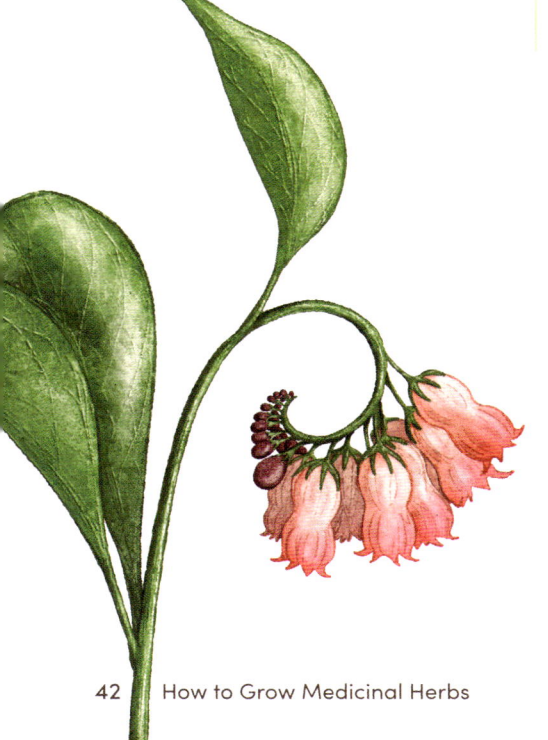

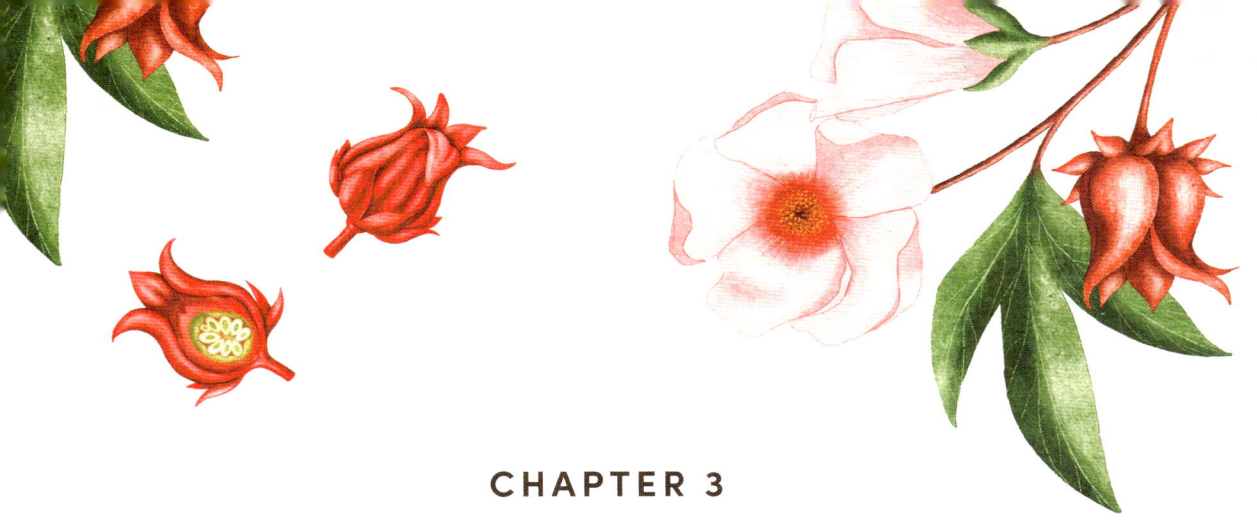

CHAPTER 3

Adding Herbs to Meals and Drinks

Capturing the magical properties of herbs doesn't just happen in your apothecary! Incorporating dried and fresh herbs into your everyday drinks, soups, and seasoning blends is a digestible way of putting your herbalism into practice.

Understanding the different applications for dried herbs versus fresh herbs for teas and culinary preparations can help you effectively take your recipes to the next level. This chapter will show you various ways to incorporate medicinal herbs into the foods you eat and drink. Whether you have an abundance of fresh herbs to use in a soup or you want to capture the essence of a peak season harvest in a delicious medicinal tea, there is a recipe to fulfill each of those needs.

Cooking with Dried versus Fresh Herbs

When properly dried, fresh herbs can lose up to 90 percent of their moisture by weight. This process also concentrates their flavor, which means that you'll need a smaller amount of dried herbs to reach the desired taste and effect.

For example, to make a cup of peppermint tea, you would need at least ¼ cup of fresh smashed peppermint leaves. But you would only need 1 tablespoon of dried leaves to make the same cup of tea. It is *technically* the same amount of plant matter, but one has the majority of the moisture removed.

Recipes for Healing Foods

You may not have considered that a bundle of fresh herbs like rosemary, thyme, sage, and oregano tossed into your pot of chicken soup is a medicinal herbal preparation, but it is! These basic herbs' volatile oils infuse the broth, giving it antimicrobial, antioxidant, and decongestant qualities. The bundle supports the immune system, helps clear the lungs, and aids digestion—making a simple pot of chicken soup a medicinal powerhouse for healing! Consider trying one of these options next time you want to infuse a dish with medicinal and flavorful herbal compounds.

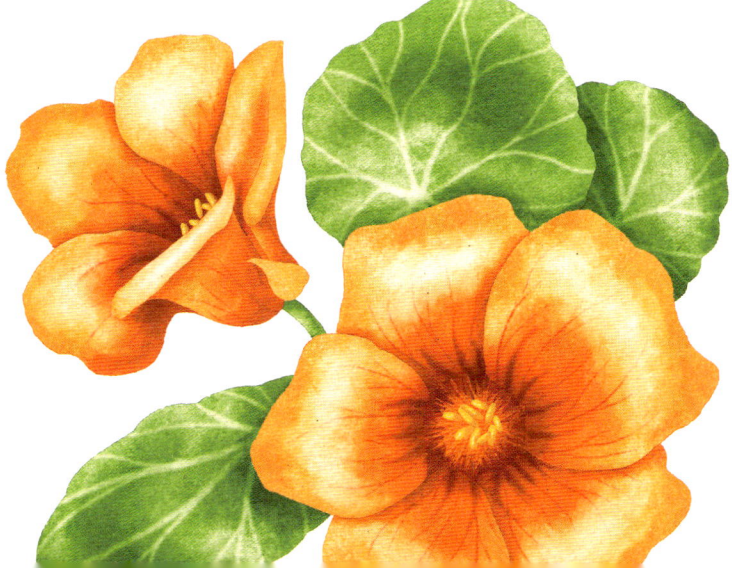

Nut-Free Nasturtium Lemon Balm Pesto

This is a peppery lemon-scented pesto alternative to the basic basil pesto. If you don't have nasturtium growing, you can substitute with peppery arugula or basil for this recipe, or use lemon balm entirely! This pesto benefits the immune system, helps relieve stress, and aids digestion. The peppery garlic and nasturtium leaves can help to warm the body and clear mucus, aiding in respiratory support along with providing antibacterial properties.

Makes 1 cup pesto

WHAT YOU'LL NEED:

1 cup fresh nasturtium leaves

1 cup fresh lemon balm leaves

1–2 garlic cloves

1 tablespoon roasted sunflower seeds

2–3 tablespoons shredded Parmesan cheese

Juice of ½–1 whole lemon, to taste

½ teaspoon salt, or to taste

⅓–½ cup olive oil, to taste/ consistency preference

WHAT TO DO:

1. Add all ingredients except olive oil to a food processor or blender. Pulse a few times to break them down. With motor running, slowly drizzle in olive oil until a smooth, spoonable paste forms.
2. Taste, and adjust lemon juice, salt, and/or oil as needed.

Ghormeh Sabzi (Persian Fried Herb Stew)

This traditional Iranian stew features vibrant flavors from the variety of aromatic herbs, onions, and fenugreek. It's a powerhouse of digestive, anti-inflammatory, and nutritive herbs. Cilantro helps calm inflammation, and fenugreek is a powerful digestive herb. With the fiber from multiple leafy herbs and kidney beans, plus the digestive support of fenugreek, this herbal stew is a great reset for a slow digestive system.

Makes 6–8 servings

WHAT YOU'LL NEED:

2 tablespoons + ¼ cup extra-virgin olive oil or neutral oil, divided

1 large white onion, diced

2 pounds beef or lamb stew meat, cut into 1" pieces

1 teaspoon ground turmeric

1 tablespoon salt, or to taste

4 cups finely chopped fresh parsley leaves

5 cups chopped fresh cilantro leaves

1 cup chopped chives or green onions

1 tablespoon dried fenugreek leaves (or 2–3 teaspoons fenugreek seeds, crushed)

1 (15-ounce) can red kidney beans, drained and rinsed

2 whole dried limes with holes poked in them (or 2 tablespoons lime juice + zest from 1 lime) plus 2 whole fresh limes for garnish

WHAT TO DO:

1. In a large pot, heat 2 tablespoons olive oil on medium heat. Once shimmering, add onion and sauté until golden. Add meat and turmeric. Sear until browned on all sides. Season with salt.

2. Add 3 cups water to cover meat. Bring to a boil, then lower heat to a simmer and cover with a lid while you prepare the herbs.

3. In a separate pan, heat ¼ cup oil. Gently "fry" parsley, cilantro, chives, and fenugreek over medium heat for 5–10 minutes, just until the greens begin to deepen in color. Reduce heat to low and stir for 10 more minutes. The herbs will turn a dark green color when ready.

4. Combine fried herbs with simmering meat mixture and add kidney beans and limes. Add a bit more water if necessary to cover entire mixture and bring to a simmer.

5. Cook until flavors combine and meat is tender but not completely falling apart, about 1 hour. Serve with additional squeeze of fresh limes over steamed white rice.

Honey Lime Cilantro Mint Vinaigrette

This sweet and refreshing tangy vinaigrette and marinade has just the right balance of flavors. You can use it to marinate meats or veggies or as a vinaigrette with raw veggies and salads. There are cooling and cleansing properties in the mint and cilantro. Plus, the lime juice, mint, garlic, and cilantro all aid in digestion, making this vinaigrette a great topping for salads and grilled meats in the summertime to increase efficient digestion of fats, raw veggies, and proteins while cooling down the body.

Makes 1 cup vinaigrette

WHAT YOU'LL NEED:

¼ cup packed fresh mint leaves

½ cup packed fresh cilantro leaves

½ cup freshly squeezed lime juice

2 tablespoons honey

1 garlic clove

Pinch of salt, or to taste

½ cup extra-virgin olive oil or neutral oil, or to consistency preference

WHAT TO DO:

1. Add everything but the olive oil to a food processor and pulse until a paste forms.
2. Drizzle in olive oil until the mixture turns into a loose dressing with your preferred consistency.

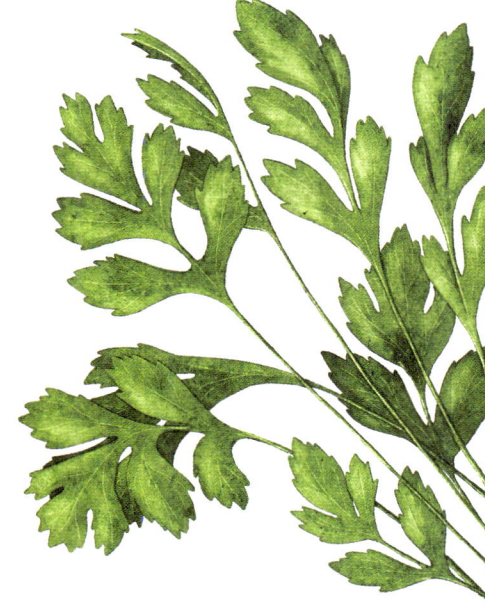

Dried Herb Seasoning Blends

Dried herbs offer concentrated flavor that can enhance everything from meats to soups to marinades. With just a few core
herbs in your garden, you can create multiple pantry staples by
utilizing the dehydration techniques you learned in Chapter 2.

Herb and Feather Seasoning

This is a medicinal and versatile herb-filled dry seasoning blend that pairs
well with poultry dishes and complements a variety of roasted vegetables as
well. Consider this an all-purpose herbal blend for everyday cooking.

Makes about ½ cup seasoning blend

WHAT YOU'LL NEED:

2 tablespoons dried sage

1 tablespoon dried thyme

1 tablespoon dried rosemary

1 tablespoon dried basil

1 tablespoon dried garlic

2 teaspoons dried oregano

1–1½ tablespoons salt, to taste

WHAT TO DO:

1. Combine all herbs and salt in a small bowl.
   Make sure your herbs and salt are a similar
   size so the seasoning mixes well.
2. Store in an airtight jar and use 1 tablespoon
   per pound of meat (or to taste) for seasoning.

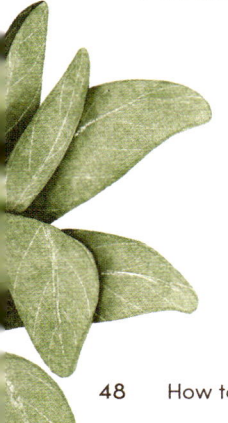

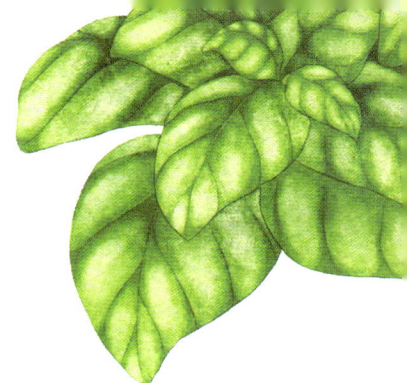

Salt Blends

Using salt to preserve herbs is a great way to make a simple flavor-filled seasoning with a large harvest of fresh herbs.

Basil Salt

Use this herb-infused salt to season meats, roasted vegetables, French fries, and popcorn. Feel free to experiment, making herbed salt with different herbs from your garden. In this version, basil is great for stimulating appetite and relieving gas and bloating. With mild nervine properties, it can also be uplifting and calming for the nervous system.

Makes ½–⅔ cups salt

WHAT YOU'LL NEED:

½ cup fresh basil leaves

½ cup salt

WHAT TO DO:

1. Wash and thoroughly dry the fresh basil leaves (moisture = mold risk).
2. Add basil and salt to a food processor or blender. Pulse until a damp, green paste forms.
3. Spread paste on a parchment-lined baking sheet and bake at 170–190°F until dry, for 30–60 minutes, stirring at least once. Or, place into a dehydrator at 95–115°F until dry, for 6–12 hours.
4. Pulse again in the food processor if large chunks remain after baking. Store in an airtight jar at room temperature for up to 6 months.

Infusing Drinks with Herbs

Brewing a proper cup of herbal tea is one of the easiest ways to consume and enjoy your medicinal herbs regularly. But tea is not the *only* way to infuse herbs into your drinks. In this section, you will learn the basics of how to brew the best cup of herbal tea, plus a few foundational herbal infusions that have been made for years throughout different cultures. You can use any of them simply as refreshing drinks, but they can also help you cool down and hydrate, and support your digestion. No fancy equipment is needed, just fresh herbs, a few pantry staples, and a bit of time to let the plants do their work!

HERBAL TEAS

To brew herbal teas for both flavor and medicinal benefit, it's important to brew them at the right temperature and to use the correct ratio of herbs to water. For teas made with leaves and flowers, like mint, lemon balm, or chamomile, it's best to use water that is between 180 and 200°F (just below a full boil, steaming strongly but not bubbling). Water that's hotter than that can destroy heat-sensitive plant components, like essential oils. Water at the proper temperature preserves aroma, color, and medicinal properties, especially in fresh herbs. Here are some additional tips:

- For the best baseline ratio of herbs to water, start with 1 tablespoon of dried herbs or ¼ cup of fresh herbs packed lightly per 1 cup of water. You can adjust this ratio based on the final flavor profile and potency you want with different herbal blends. In Part 2, each herb profile will give a more specific suggested measurement of herb amounts per cup of tea. Steep anywhere from 10–20 minutes depending on your preference.
- Some medicinal herbs have strong grassy or bitter flavors, so incorporating them in smaller amounts alongside dried fruits or sweeter-tasting herbs can help you have a palatable yet powerful combination to enjoy.
- Be sure you always cover your teacup or jar to trap in essential oils that otherwise might evaporate.

Consider trying out the following tea blends for both herbal support and flavor.

Blueberry Mint Hibiscus Cooler

This tea is a refreshing way to cool down in hot weather. Plus, hibiscus can help lower blood pressure, and the mint promotes cooling through menthol. To enjoy this drink hot, consider replacing the mint with ginger. You can serve this chilled with a squeeze of fresh orange or lime, or make a concentrated batch using half of the water, then top with sparkling water for a spritzer.

Makes 2 cups concentrate, 1 quart cooler

WHAT YOU'LL NEED:

¼ cup dried hibiscus petals

1 tablespoon dried mint

1 teaspoon dried lemon balm

2 tablespoons dried holy basil

1 teaspoon dried rose petals

2 tablespoons dried blueberries

4 cups water, divided

1 teaspoon dried stevia leaf or sweetener of choice (optional)

WHAT TO DO:

1. Combine dried herbs in a quart-sized Mason jar. Bring 2 cups of water to just below a boil (180–200°F) and pour over the dried herbs. Place a covering over the tea to contain the volatile oils while steeping. Let steep for 10 minutes, then strain the herbs from the brewed tea.

2. **For a concentrate:** If you opt to use this tea as a concentrate (to add into other drinks, like sparkling water), let the 2 cups of prepared mixture cool down to room temperature first, then refrigerate to chill fully for 3–4 hours. To use this concentrate, start with a ratio of 1 part sparkling or still water to 1 part concentrate.

3. **Ready-to-drink ratio:** If you want to drink this entire recipe at the intended ratio as a chilled, ready-to-drink preparation, add 2 cups of cold water to the 2 cups of brewed tea, and let the entire mixture cool for 30 minutes on the counter. Pour over ice and enjoy!

4. This tea can be stored for 3–5 days safely in the refrigerator as both a concentrate or a fully diluted mixture. The addition of sweeteners can expedite spoilage, so when preparing larger batches of tea to drink for a few days, sweeten as you prepare each serving.

Soothing Catnip Chamomile Tea

This blend of soothing herbs is just what you need to calm anxiety and get better sleep. Start out by drinking a small cup in the evening to see how it affects you. If the flavor is too bitter or grassy, sweeten with honey and add a squeeze of fresh lemon juice. A teaspoon or two of dried apple pieces will sweeten this blend as well and bring out the notes of the chamomile and lemon balm.

Makes one 10–12-ounce cup tea

WHAT YOU'LL NEED:

½ teaspoon dried passion vine

2 teaspoons dried lemon balm

½ teaspoon dried catnip

1 tablespoon dried chamomile

1–2 teaspoons dried apples (to sweeten this blend and bring out the notes of chamomile and lemon balm; optional)

WHAT TO DO:

Combine all ingredients in a large mug, cover with 10–12 ounces hot but not boiling water (180–200°F), and let steep for 15 minutes. Place a cover over this tea while steeping to contain the volatile oils. Strain the herbs from the brewed tea and enjoy!

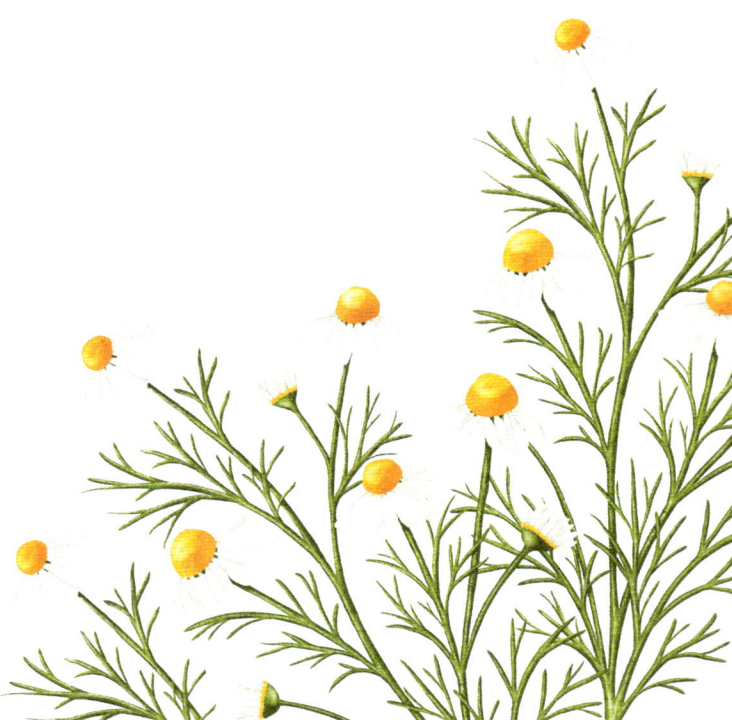

Breathe Deep
Cold and Flu Support Tea

This is a base blend of herbs that can open the lungs for deeper breathing, help induce sweating, cool down a fever, and support the immune system. Treating the symptoms of an acute infection requires a tailored approach for the specific symptoms you want to reduce, so you might consider subtracting or adding different herbs to make a custom blend in small batches. The mint soothes digestion and relieves nausea, while the yarrow helps manage fevers and provides acute cold/flu support. The echinacea will help boost the immune system, while elderberry is rich in vitamin C. Sweeten this blend with honey if you like. Note: Elderberry will become bitter if steeped for long periods.

Makes one 10–12-ounce cup tea

WHAT YOU'LL NEED:

2 teaspoons dried mint

1 teaspoon dried yarrow flowers/leaves

1–2 teaspoons dried echinacea flowers/leaves

2 teaspoons dried elderberry

WHAT TO DO:

Combine all ingredients in a large mug, cover with 10–12 ounces hot but not boiling water (180–200°F), and let steep for 10 minutes. Place a cover over this tea while steeping to contain the volatile oils. Strain herbs from the brewed tea and enjoy.

This base recipe can support the typical complaints from someone struggling with cold and flu symptoms, but consider the following additions or substitutions to support the body in dealing with specific symptoms. This is when having your own apothecary stocked with herbs can really come in handy!

- If the person feels chilled, sluggish, or has body aches without heat, choose ginger, which is warming and stimulating.
- If the person has nausea *and* is chilled, you can swap out the mint in this base recipe with 1 teaspoon of dried ginger or a ¼"-thick slice of fresh ginger, as both mint and ginger help with nausea but have different energetics.
- If the person suffers from dry skin or a dry, scratchy throat or dry cough, consider pairing mint or ginger with a moistening herb, like licorice root or mullein.
- If the person needs to moisten dry respiratory tissue, soothe irritation, or loosen stuck mucus, add 1–2 teaspoons of dried mullein to this base blend. (Make sure to strain tea made with loose-leaf mullein using a cheesecloth or fine-mesh sieve, because this herb has a lot of tiny little hairs on the leaves that can irritate.)
- If the person needs to coat the throat and lungs, you can add ½ teaspoon of licorice root to this blend. (It also adds sweetness.)

DECOCTIONS

To extract the most medicinal compounds from tougher plant parts, like roots, seeds, and bark (such as ginger, dandelion root, echinacea root, or licorice), you'll want to make a stronger infusion called a "decoction." To make a decoction, you can simmer the parts gently in water for 15–30 minutes, then strain. Always use a lid while simmering to preserve volatile oils.

If using dried herbs, use about 1 tablespoon of herbs per 1 cup of water. Use a higher ratio of herbs if you are aiming for stronger therapeutic strength. If using fresh herbs, use about ¼ cup of herbs per 1 cup of water.

NOTE: For medicinal tea blends that contain both leafy herbs and tougher roots, you can let the entire blend steep for a few minutes longer or make a separate decoction of the roots and keep it stored in small batches in the fridge for up to 2 days. Then warm up the decoction along with the other herbs in the tea blends for peak medicinal potency.

ACCOUNTING FOR TANNINS

Some herbs, like yarrow, blue vervain, and self-heal, contain tannins, which are astringent, polyphenolic compounds. They have a drying or puckering effect and are helpful for tightening tissues, toning mucous membranes, and reducing inflammation, both internally and externally.

When brewing herbs with tannins in teas or decoctions, it's important to note that the longer these herbs are steeped, the more bitter those tannins can become.

Sometimes you're brewing them for a necessary use and the taste is a secondary concern. But if you are more focused on the overall flavor of your brews, it's best to know which herbs have tannins so you don't steep them for too long.

Oxymels

WHAT ARE OXYMELS?

Oxymels are a vinegar and raw honey compound that can be blended with medicinal herbs to deliver them in a delicious and easy-to-take form. The word comes from the ancient Greek combination of *oxy* (meaning "acid") and *meli* (meaning "honey"), and the remedy is old, originating in Persia and Greece. Making herbal remedies that actually taste good can be a challenge sometimes because strongly flavored medicinal herbs can take over the flavor profile, but oxymels solve that problem. Plus, honey and vinegar combined can help with respiratory issues, digestion, sore throats, and fever reduction even without the addition of herbs.

WHAT TYPES OF HERBS ARE BEST FOR OXYMELS?

Herbal combinations that work well in oxymels include:

- Sage and thyme for viral flu and stomach issues.
- Marshmallow root and ginger for coughs and congestions.
- Dandelion root for liver support, bile production, and appetite.
- St.-John's-wort for mood support.

HOW TO MAKE A BASIC OXYMEL

To make the base of an oxymel, mix 1 part vinegar and 1 part honey. You'll then pour the mixture over the herbs you're including to completely cover them before placing in a glass jar. Cap the jar tightly with plastic or wax paper under a metal lid to prevent corrosion. Steep in a cool dark place for 2–4 weeks. Strain.

Keep in mind that an oxymel does not have to always be a 50:50 ratio, so feel free to reduce or increase the honey if it helps make the mixture more palatable for you.

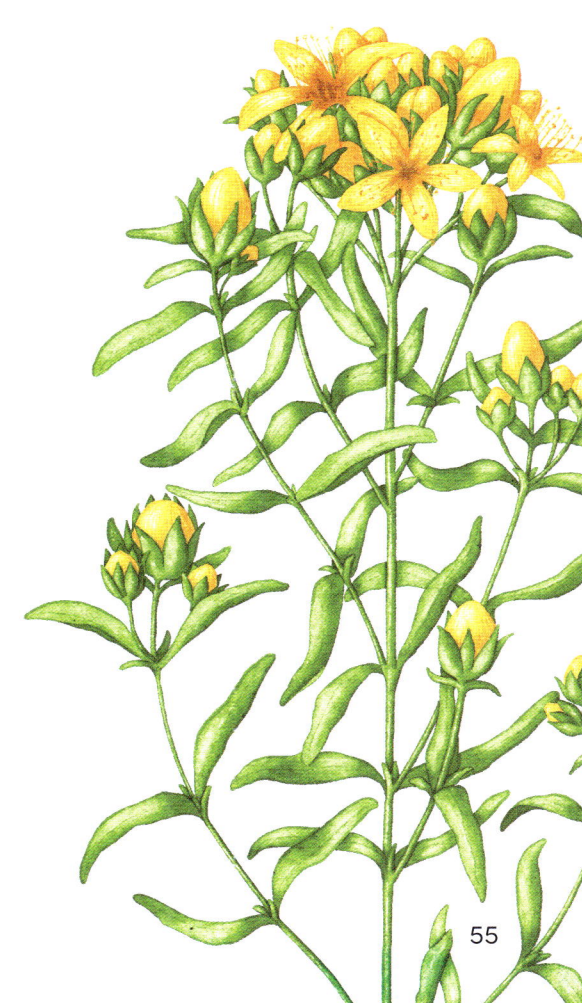

Fire Cider

Often used in the winter months to help ward off colds, aid in decongestion, and increase digestive support, fire cider is a common oxymel. It is often on the savory side, using additions like onions, garlic, and pungent herbs. If the hot peppers are too much for you, omit them. But adding honey can make taking mouthfuls of this mixture a lot more palatable.

Makes about 3 cups strained cider

WHAT YOU'LL NEED:

1 cup garlic cloves, peeled and chopped

½ white or yellow onion, cut into large chunks

½ cup freshly grated horseradish

2–3 fresh hot peppers (like jalapeño or cayenne), sliced

2 cups apple cider vinegar

1 cup raw honey, or to taste

OPTIONAL INGREDIENTS:

1 cup freshly grated ginger

2 tablespoons freshly grated turmeric

2–3 sprigs fresh rosemary

½ fresh lemon, sliced

½ fresh orange, sliced

1 teaspoon ground cinnamon

Other medicinal herbs of your choosing

WHAT TO DO:

1. Place garlic, onion, horseradish, hot peppers, and any optional ingredients in a clean quart-sized jar.
2. Pour apple cider vinegar over ingredients until they are fully covered, leaving 1–2" at the top. Cover with a plastic lid or line a metal lid with parchment, as the metal can corrode.
3. Store jar in a cool, dark place for 3–4 weeks, shaking daily to help the extraction.
4. Strain through cheesecloth or a fine-mesh sieve into a clean jar.
5. Stir in raw honey to taste.

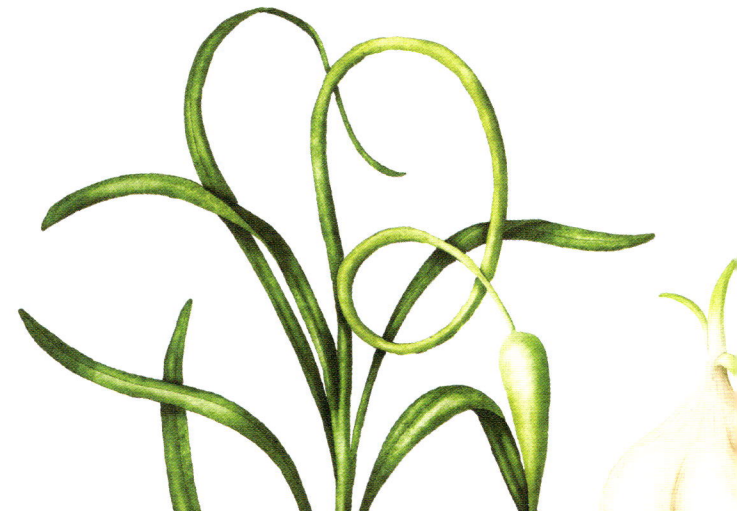

For best use, consume fire cider in small, regular doses, since it's both strong in flavor and potent medicinally. Here are some of the best ways to regularly consume this herbal remedy:

- **Straight from the spoon:** Take 1 tablespoon daily as a preventative tonic during cold and flu season. At the first sign of a cold or flu, increase to 1 tablespoon every 3–4 hours.
- **Dilute in water or tea:** Mix 1 tablespoon in a cup of warm water or herbal tea. This reduces the intensity while still delivering medicinal benefits. This is especially useful for people with acid reflux or a stomach sensitivity.
- **With honey:** Stir 1 tablespoon of fire cider into 1 teaspoon of raw honey for a throat-soothing, immune-supporting remedy.
- **As food medicine:** Use as a salad dressing base and mix with oil at a ratio of 1 part fire cider (vinegar) to 3 parts oil of choice (olive oil is a great option). Additionally, you can whisk in 1 teaspoon of mustard for a creamier base and to add balance for salads.

Keep in mind that fire cider is very pungent and acidic, so it is not always tolerated well on an empty stomach. With the base of this recipe being vinegar, consuming large amounts of fire cider daily for long periods of time can stress tooth enamel and digestion.

Herbal Elixirs

WHAT ARE HERBAL ELIXIRS?

Herbal elixirs are similar to oxymels, but an elixir can use different types of sweeteners, while oxymels *only* use honey. An elixir is a sweet, alcohol-based herbal preparation that combines the potency of a tincture with the flavor and soothing qualities of honey or syrup. Some elixirs do use honey, but they can also use sweeteners like cane sugar, molasses, and maple syrup.

WHAT TYPES OF HERBS ARE BEST FOR HERBAL ELIXIRS?

These herbs are often used in herbal elixirs:

- **Aromatic/sweet-tasting herbs:** Lavender, anise hyssop, rose petals, mint, and lemon balm.
- **Nervine/adaptogenic herbs:** Holy basil, lemon balm, chamomile, St.-John's-wort, catnip, passion vine, milky oats, and skullcap.
- **Circulatory or heart tonic herbs:** Rose petals, thyme, rosemary, sage, yarrow, and roselle hibiscus.
- **Immune supportive herbs:** Elderberry, elderflower, echinacea, calendula, thyme, and holy basil.

HOW TO MAKE A BASIC HERBAL ELIXIR

To make the base of an herbal elixir, mix 2 parts tincture to 1 part honey or sweetener of choice.

Herbal Syrups

WHAT ARE HERBAL SYRUPS?

Another tasty herbal preparation for medicinal herbs is herbal syrups. Herbal syrups consist of a water infusion (tea) or decoction (stronger infusion) strained and mixed with honey or another sweetener. Herbal syrups are popular for use with children due to their palatable nature.

WHAT TYPES OF HERBS ARE BEST FOR HERBAL SYRUPS?

These herbs work well in herbal syrups:

- **Immunity herbs:** Elderberry, elderflower, echinacea, yarrow (steeped for shorter amounts of time due to tannins), and holy basil.
- **Respiratory herbs:** Mullein, licorice, marshmallow, horehound, and elecampane.
- **Calming digestive herbs:** Chamomile, lemon balm, anise hyssop, rose, and lavender.

HOW TO MAKE A BASIC HERBAL SYRUP

To make the base of an herbal syrup, steep herbs in 4 cups of water for 30–45 minutes until decoction has reduced by half. Let cool, then strain and mix with 2 cups of raw honey. Syrups that are a 1:1 ratio of herbal decoction to honey/sugar can be safely stored in the fridge for about 1 month. Extra-sweet syrups with a ratio of 2 parts sweetener to 1 part herbal decoction can be stored safely in the fridge for 3–6 months.

Elderberry Syrup Recipe

This is a popular herbal syrup preparation that can help support the immune system when the first onset of viral symptoms occurs. The cinnamon, cloves, and ginger are warming, while the elderberry adds antioxidants.

Makes about 2 cups

WHAT YOU'LL NEED:

1 cup dried elderberries (or 2 cups fresh)

4 cups water

1–2 cinnamon sticks

4–6 slices fresh ginger

3–4 whole cloves

1 cup raw honey

WHAT TO DO:

1. In a medium pot, combine everything except the honey. Bring to a gentle boil, then reduce to a simmer.
2. Simmer uncovered for 30–45 minutes, until liquid has reduced by about half. Mash berries gently with a spoon to release more juice.
3. Strain through a fine-mesh sieve or cheesecloth into a glass measuring cup. You should have about 1 cup of elderberry decoction left. (If more, simmer longer; if less, top with a little hot water.)
4. While the liquid is still warm (not hot), stir in raw honey for a 1:1 ratio of sweetener to herbal decoction. Mix until sweetener is fully dissolved.
5. Pour into a sterilized glass jar or bottle. The syrup will keep for 2–3 months in the fridge.

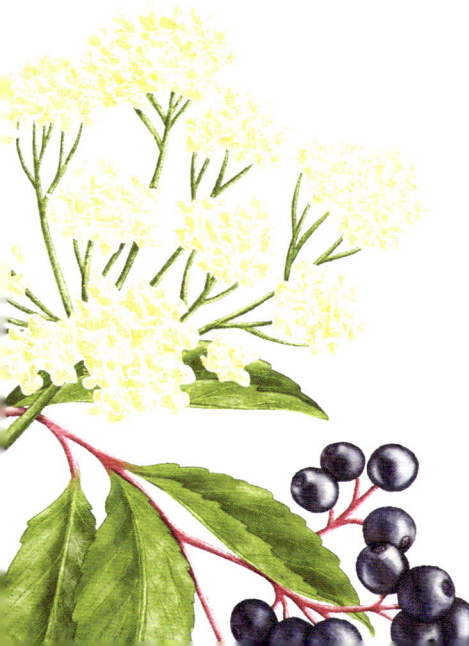

Switchels

WHAT IS A SWITCHEL?

A switchel is a tangy and sweet vinegar-based drink made with water, a natural sweetener (like honey or maple syrup), and ginger. It's sometimes called "haymaker's punch" because it was popular among eighteenth- and nineteenth-century farmers as a natural electrolyte drink during hot fieldwork. Switchels can also be a great energizing alternative to a caffeine-based drink and can help support the body's ability to cool down or increase digestion before or after heavy meals.

Switchels are endlessly customizable. You can steep herbs directly in the water used for the base of the switchel to infuse even more medicinal properties into this drink or use herb-infused vinegars and syrups as a base.

WHAT TYPES OF HERBS ARE BEST FOR SWITCHELS?

Herbs that are great for cooling and soothing in a switchel are mint, lemon balm, rose petals, lavender, and roselle hibiscus. Warming herbs that can support digestion in a switchel are ginger, cinnamon (a spice), lemongrass, rosemary, and holy basil (aka tulsi).

HOW TO MAKE A BASIC SWITCHEL

Here's a fruity and soothing switchel recipe.

Strawberry Tulsi Ginger Switchel

This switchel can support the body when under physical and emotional stress, aid in digestion, boost the natural process of sweating to cool down, and even gently energize. The macerated strawberries in this recipe can give some texture to the base of the drink, but you can strain out the berry solids from the honey and the berry juice that forms during the maceration process before combining with the herbal decoction if you prefer a less pulpy drink.

This recipe makes 2 cups concentrate that can be diluted into 4 cups of a large, ready-to-drink batch

WHAT YOU'LL NEED:

1–1½ cups fresh sliced strawberries

1½–2 tablespoons honey or maple syrup

4 tablespoons dried tulsi (holy basil) or 1½ cups fresh tulsi leaves, loosely packed

2 tablespoons grated fresh ginger (add an extra tablespoon if you like spicy ginger flavor)

2½ cups water

1½ tablespoons raw apple cider vinegar

OPTIONAL INGREDIENTS:

2 cups cold water (for full-quart batch)

Ice cubes

Sparkling water

Sea salt

Squeeze of lemon or lime

WHAT TO DO:

1. First, macerate the strawberries: In a 2-quart pitcher or jar, combine sliced strawberries with honey or maple syrup. Mash lightly and let sit to extract the juice from the berries.

2. Now, make a decoction: In a small pot, combine tulsi and ginger with water. Simmer gently, lid ajar, for 10–15 minutes. The liquid amount should be reduced by about ½ cup.

3. Turn heat to low, cover the pot fully, and steep for another 10 minutes. Strain the herbs from this decoction using a fine-mesh strainer or cheesecloth.

4. Pour the warm, not hot (100–115°F), decoction over the macerated strawberry-honey mixture. Stir well and let cool to room temperature. Add apple cider vinegar and stir well to combine.

5. This combination is now the concentrate (base) for your switchel. You can chill this for 3–4 hours in the fridge to dilute later, or you can dilute it immediately to serve.

6. To make a full-quart (4-cup) batch of ready-to-drink switchel, add 2 cups of cold water to the 2 cups of switchel concentrate and stir. Serve immediately and enjoy. This mixture can be stored safely in the fridge for 2–3 days.

7. To make an effervescent switchel with this concentrate, simply add ½–¾ cup of switchel concentrate to a 12-ounce glass, top with a few ice cubes, and fill the glass the rest of the way with sparkling water. Sea salt or a fresh squeeze of lemon or lime can amplify the electrolyte benefits.

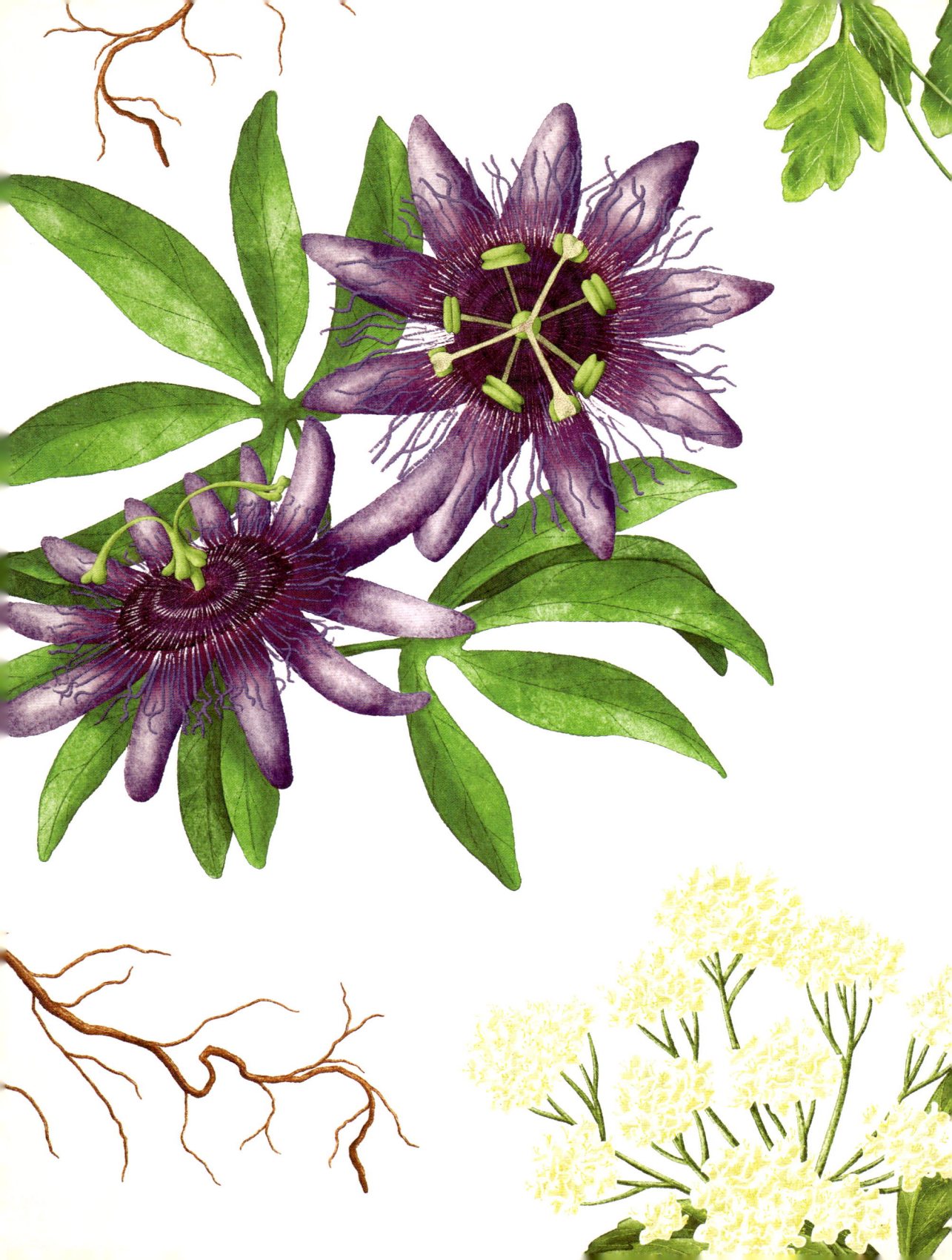

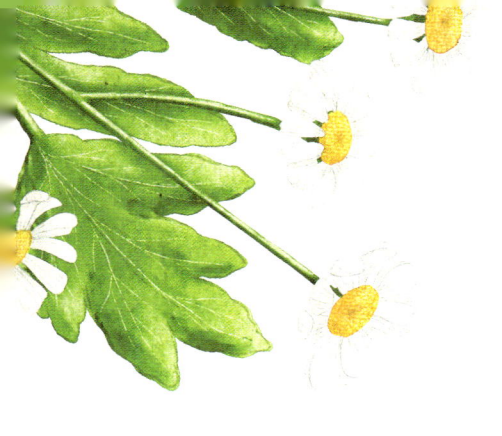
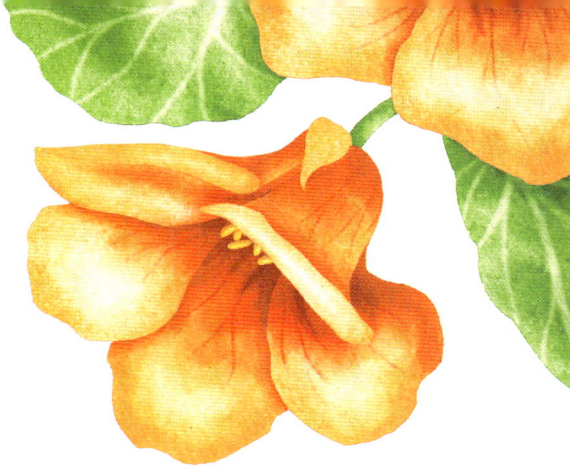

PART 2

Medicinal Herbs

In this part, you'll find in-depth profiles of fifty common medicinal herbs, along with an illustration of how the plant looks. You'll learn each plant's medicinal properties and the basics of planting that herb, including how to sow seeds, space plants, and determine what type of soil to cultivate. Then you'll find a list of common ways to use that herb, from teas to tinctures to poultices. The wealth of information here will help maintain your well-being, inside and out, in a natural way.

Terms to Know

Here are some key words you'll see used in the herb profiles to describe herbal properties and solutions:

- **Adaptogen:** Helps the body adapt to stress.
- **Analgesic:** Relieves pain.
- **Antifungal:** Prevents fungal growth.
- **Antimicrobial:** Inhibits growth of microorganisms.
- **Antiseptic:** Prevents bacteria growth.
- **Antispasmodic:** Relieves or prevents muscle spasms and cramps.
- **Bitter tonic:** Stimulates digestion by triggering the bitter receptors on the tongue, which reflexively increase saliva, stomach acid, bile, and enzyme production.
- **Carminative:** Relieves gas, bloating, and digestive discomfort.
- **Demulcent:** Soothes irritation or inflammation.
- **Diaphoretic:** Encourages perspiration to support the body's natural cooling process.
- **Diuretic:** Increases urine production and helps the body eliminate excess water and salts through the kidneys.
- **Emollient:** Soothes skin.
- **Emmenagogue:** Stimulates menstrual flow.
- **Expectorant:** Helps clear mucus.
- **Galactagogue:** Supports lactation.
- **Lymphagogue:** Helps detoxify.
- **Nervine:** Supports the nervous system, calming anxiety and restlessness or gently stimulating when fatigue is present.

Each herb profile that follows also describes topical and internal safety information for that herb. Here are some additional safety guidelines to keep in mind:

- You should always speak to a health-care professional who knows your individual circumstances before using any herbs, topically or internally.
- For topical treatments, always test the solution on a small patch of skin before using more extensively.
- While some herbs are considered safe for pregnant or nursing women, limited research exists on the topic, so check with your healthcare provider in this and other special circumstances.
- Check with a veterinarian before using herbs with animals.

Anise Hyssop

Agastache foeniculum

Short-lived perennial in zones 4–9, variety dependent

This perennial member of the mint family has fragrant, licorice-scented leaves and tall spikes of purple flowers that attract pollinators.

Medicinal Properties:

TOPICAL: Mild antimicrobial that soothes minor burns, scrapes, and skin irritations.

INTERNAL: Carminative that aids in sluggish digestion; mild expectorant that soothes irritated throats and chest congestion, and supports recovery from respiratory infections; gentle nervine and mild diaphoretic.

ENERGETIC: Slightly warming, drying.

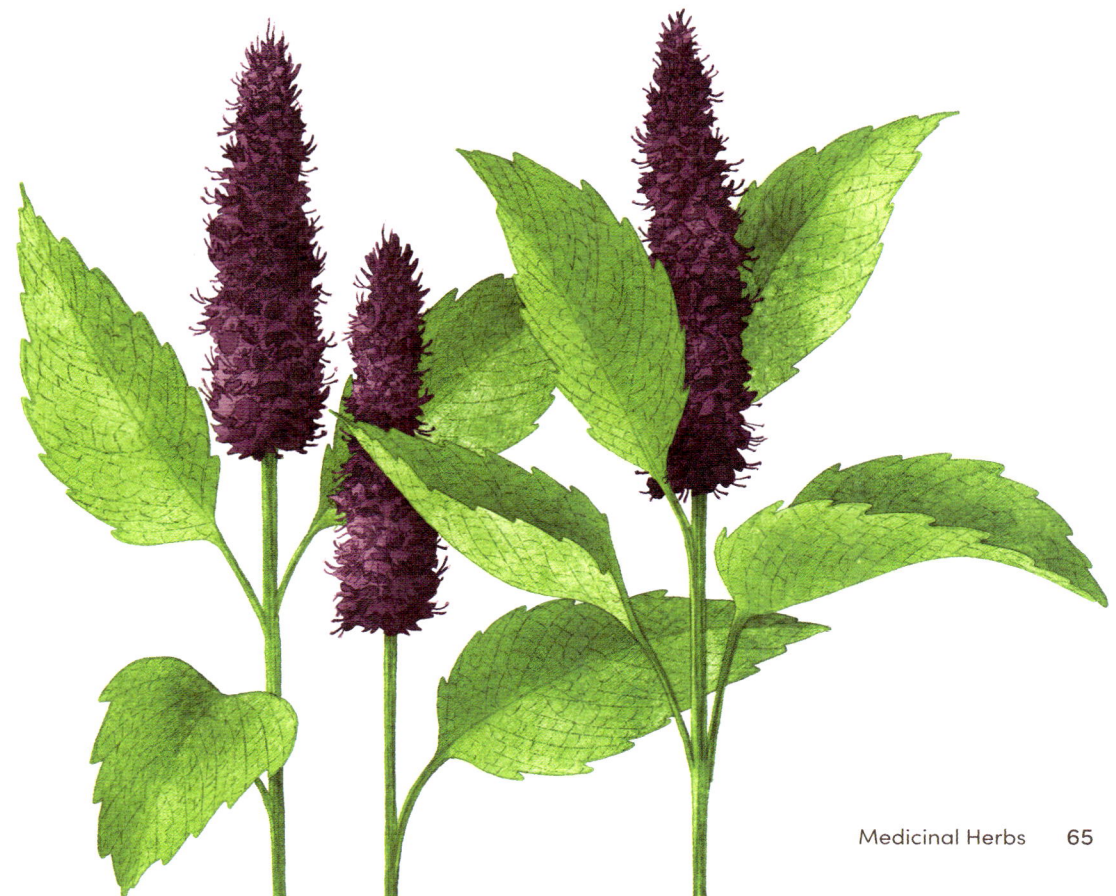

How to Grow:

 WHEN TO PLANT: Sow or transplant after the danger of frost has passed. In mild climates, start seeds indoors 6–8 weeks before last frost.

 GROWS BEST FROM: Seed, transplant, or propagation. Seeds do better with cold stratification. Sow seeds on the soil surface and gently press in. Keep soil moist and warm for better germination. Seeds need light to germinate. Germination can take 10–15 days. Direct sowing may be difficult because the seeds are tiny. Anise hyssop easily propagates in water or soil. Divide established clumps in spring or fall.

 SUN AND SOIL NEEDS: Full sun, 6–8 hours or more, but tolerates partial shade. Needs well-drained, moderately rich soil. Regular watering is preferred, but established plants can tolerate some drought with good mulch practices.

 VARIETIES TO TRY: Straight species, Golden Jubilee, Blue Fortune, Black Adder, Korean mint, and Mexican hyssop.

 SPACING: Space plants 12–18" apart. Anise hyssop grows more vertical than wide, but it can spread through rhizomes (similar to other mint varieties), so plan accordingly. Container friendly.

 BLOOM TIME: 60–90 days from seed to initial small harvest; 90–100 days from seed when plants are well established. Produces flowers in the summer.

 HARVESTING TIPS: Begin harvesting leaves once plants are at least 8–12" tall. The best flavor and potency is just before plants start to flower. If you need usable leaves sooner, start mint from cuttings or divisions. You can harvest within 4–6 weeks instead of waiting 2–3 months from seed.

GROWING TIP:

Anise hyssop is not a true hyssop, but it belongs to the mint family. It is considered a short-lived perennial because healthy new growth can slow down after 3–5 years, but it reseeds easily, allowing a continuous cycle of healthy growth.

How to Use:

 INFUSED OIL: Oil infusions are best made with dried leaves and flowers.

 TINCTURE: 1 part fresh aerial parts (flowers, stems, and leaves) to 2 parts 40–50% alcohol, or 1 part dried leaves to 5 parts 40–50% alcohol. Tincture can be used as an expectorant and a demulcent.

 TEA: Steep 1 tablespoon dried leaves and flowers, or ¼ cup fresh leaves and flowers, per 1 cup hot water, covered, for 5–10 minutes. These teas can help soothe cough, congestion, and sore throats, and relieve gas and bloating.

 POULTICE AND COMPRESS: A warm poultice may be used on the chest for mild congestion relief. A cool compress can be placed over the forehead or neck to ease tension headaches or mild fevers.

〳〳〳 **STEAM INHALATION:** Add a handful of fresh leaves, or 2–3 tablespoons dried leaves, to a bowl of hot water. Tent your head with a towel and inhale vapors for 5–10 minutes to help open airways and calm dry, hacking coughs or lingering bronchial irritation.

⚠ General Safety:

TOPICAL USE: Generally safe on skin, but test first and dilute when needed. Avoid use on broken skin or long-term use without guidance.

INTERNAL USE: Generally safe in tea and medicinal use. Limited research exists, but hyssop has a long history of safe culinary use for pregnant and nursing women.

HERBALIST TIP:

Anise hyssop is so beneficial for attracting and supporting pollinators that you should always plant more than you need to support them!

Bacopa

Bacopa monnieri

Annual in most zones, tender perennial in tropical climates

This is a creeping, water-loving herb with small succulent leaves and delicate white to lavender flowers. It's often valued for supporting memory, focus, and nervous system health.

Medicinal Properties:

TOPICAL: Anti-inflammatory, skin-soothing properties.

INTERNAL: Adaptogen and nervine that supports cognitive function and thyroid balance; anti-inflammatory.

ENERGETIC: Cooling, slightly moistening.

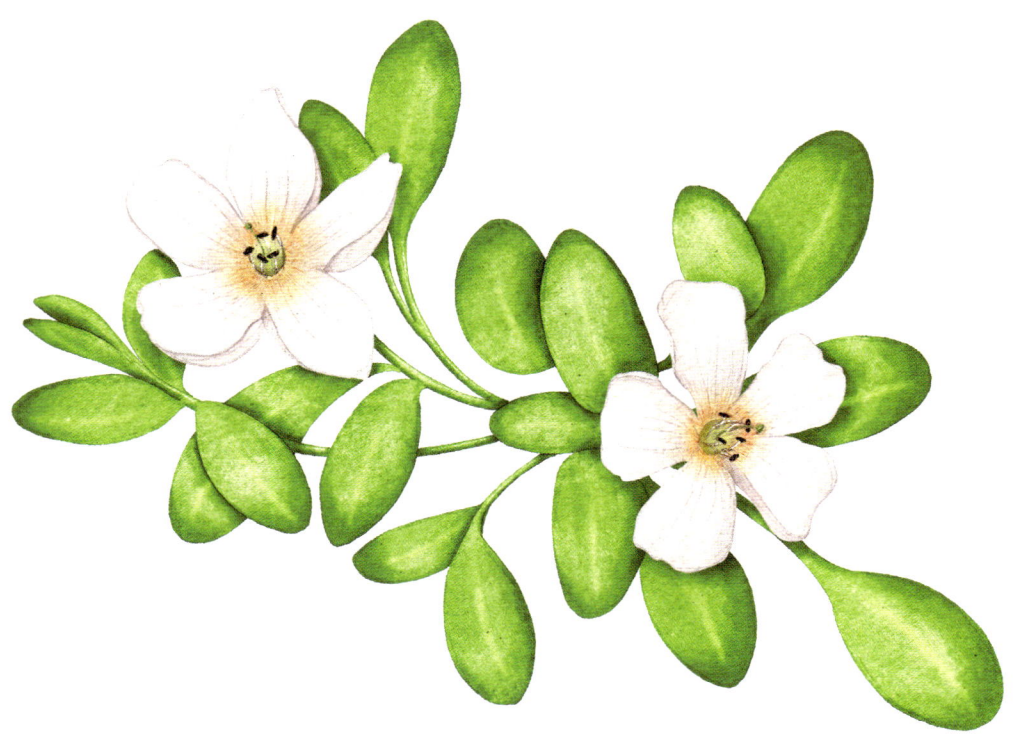

How to Grow:

 WHEN TO PLANT: Best started from cuttings or nursery plants in spring after the danger of frost has passed. Seeds are difficult to germinate but can be started 3–4 weeks before your last frost in mild climates. Bacopa is a subtropical plant and prefers warm soil. Wait to transplant outside until soil temps have reached 70°F for Bacopa to thrive.

 GROWS BEST FROM: Transplant or rooted cuttings. The seeds are very fine, almost like dust. Bacopa requires light to germinate, so try pressing seeds onto the soil surface without covering. The seeds must never dry out, so a cover or humidity dome is required for successful germination. Germination can take 2–3 weeks but sometimes up to 4–6 weeks. Cuttings can be taken from nonwoody stems and rooted in water. Once established, the root system of the plant can be dug up and divided to get more plants.

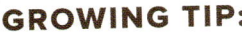

GROWING TIP:

Bacopa thrives in wet soils and even in shallow water, making it a great herb for pond edges, rain gardens, or containers kept moist.

 SUN AND SOIL NEEDS: Full sun to partial shade. Bacopa likes consistently wet soil or shallow water—perfect for ponds, bog gardens, well-watered containers, or lower areas of the garden.

 VARIETIES TO TRY: *Bacopa monnieri* and *Bacopa caroliniana*.

 SPACING: Space plants 6–12" apart or closer if using as a spreading ground cover. In water gardens, allow it to trail naturally. Container friendly.

 BLOOM TIME: Rooted stems are ready to harvest in 2–3 months once the plant has spread. From seed, this plant can take up to 6 months to establish. It produces small, pale flowers through the warm growing season (spring through summer), though flowers are not the main medicinal part.

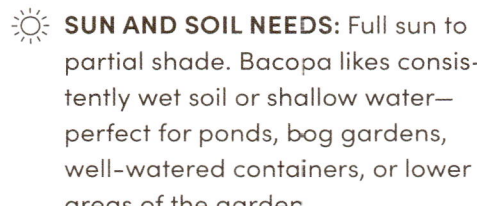 **HARVESTING TIPS:** Harvest once the plant is well established with plenty of leafy growth, usually when stems are 6–8" long and have branched out. This usually happens when the plants are at least 6–8 weeks old. Clip fresh leaves and stems as needed, leaving the plant to regrow.

How to Use:

 INFUSED OIL: Dried aerial parts can be infused into skin-safe oils to support hair growth and skin soothing.

 TINCTURE: 1 part fresh aerial parts (flowers, stems, and leaves) to 2 parts 65–70% alcohol (preferred), or 1 part dried leaves to 5 parts 40–50% alcohol. Provides concentrated relief for digestive upset and tension headaches.

 TEA: Steep 1–2 teaspoons dried, or 1 tablespoon fresh aerial parts per 1 cup hot water for 10–15 minutes to help support mental clarity and focus and calm the mind. The taste is bitter, so Bacopa is often blended with sweeter herbs.

 POULTICE AND COMPRESS: Crushed fresh leaves can be applied as a poultice for minor wounds, insect bites, or burns. A cool compress can be used to soothe rashes, inflamed itchy skin, and sunburns.

⚠ General Safety:

TOPICAL USE: Generally safe when diluted and applied to skin, but that's not a typical use for this herb. Rarely, some people may develop contact dermatitis or itchiness.

INTERNAL USE: Well tolerated in small to moderate doses in typical tincture or capsule amounts. Nausea, dry mouth, stomach cramps, diarrhea, or fatigue are possible side effects in sensitive individuals or at higher doses. May increase thyroid hormone (T3, T4) levels, so caution is advised for those with hyperthyroidism or those taking thyroid medication. Bacopa also has mild sedative and vasodilating properties, which could enhance the effects of blood pressure–lowering drugs, leading to dizziness or hypotension. Not recommended during pregnancy or nursing due to lack of safety studies.

HERBALIST TIP:

Capsules are a very common preparation for this herb, to support memory and concentration. To make a capsule, grind fully dehydrated herbs in a coffee grinder or blender. This powder can be mixed into warm water, milk, or smoothies for daily consumption, or added to capsules for ease of daily consumption as well. The typical daily dosage of powdered Bacopa is 1–3 grams of powder daily. Bacopa works best when consumed consistently over weeks or months, rather than as a one-time remedy. Pairing it with adaptogens, like holy basil, can round out its effects on memory and stress.

Basil

Ocimum basilicum
Annual

A fragrant leafy herb with lush green or purple foliage, basil is beloved in kitchens worldwide and also valued for its uplifting, digestive, and antimicrobial properties. It brings both culinary joy and medicinal support, making it a staple in herb gardens.

Medicinal Properties:

TOPICAL: Soothes insect bites, minor cuts, or acne due to its antimicrobial properties.

INTERNAL: Traditionally used to ease digestion, bloating, nausea, and poor appetite; mild calming properties; also supports the immune system.

ENERGETIC: Warming, drying.

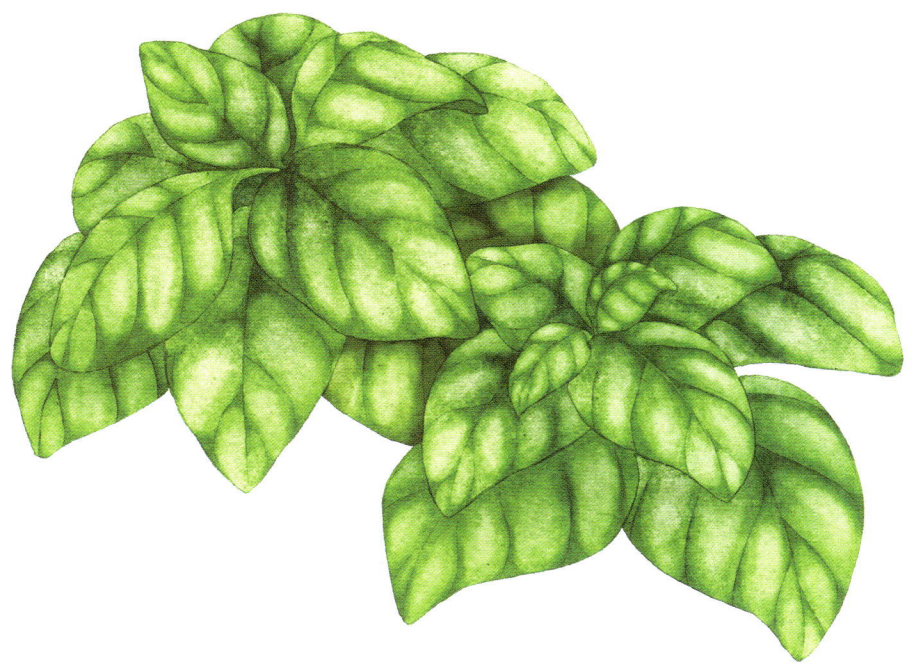

How to Grow:

 WHEN TO PLANT: Direct sow after the danger of frost has passed, when soil is consistently warm, or start inside 4–6 weeks before your last frost for transplanting. Sowing basil multiple times throughout the growing season can help you maintain a fresh supply of healthy, strong plants throughout the active growing season.

 GROWS BEST FROM: Seed or transplant. Basil is very easy to germinate and grow. It does well directly sown—press seeds lightly onto the surface of the soil and keep moist for a few weeks. You can grow it inside on a windowsill or under grow lights to transplant outside once nights have warmed up.

 SUN AND SOIL NEEDS: Full sun to partial shade. In hotter summer climates, some afternoon shade can help your basil stay tastier longer instead of wilting or bolting and going to seed. Prefers consistent moisture in well-draining soil supplemented well with organic matter.

 VARIETIES TO TRY: Genovese basil, Thai basil, holy basil, purple basil, lemon basil, and lime basil.

 SPACING: Space plants 10–12" apart. Allow 18" between rows or within containers for airflow and harvesting. Container friendly.

 BLOOM TIME: Typically 50–70 days from seed to harvest.

 HARVESTING TIPS: Basil is grown for its leaves, so harvest often before flowering. If allowed to bloom, flowers will attract pollinators but slow leaf production. Harvest once plants are 6–8" tall. Pinch just above leaf nodes (the sections of the stem where leaves grow from) to encourage branching.

GROWING TIP:

Basil is very frost sensitive, so even cool nights below 50°F can slow or damage growth. Pinching off flower buds and branches halfway up the stem can help grow bigger, healthier basil plants.

How to Use:

 INFUSED OIL: Use fresh basil leaves for infusing culinary oils or skin applications. (Ensure leaves are wilted first to avoid spoilage.)

 TINCTURE: 1 part fresh herb to 2 parts 50–60% alcohol, or 1 part dried herb to 5 parts 40–50% alcohol. Used to reduce gas and bloating and stimulate digestion and as an uplifting nervine to help clear a tired or heavy mind.

 TEA: Steep 1–2 teaspoons dried leaves, or 1–2 tablespoons fresh leaves, per 1 cup hot water, covered, for 10–15 minutes. This tea is helpful for relieving gas and bloating, easing mild stomach cramps and colic, stimulating appetite and digestion, and mild stress relief.

 POULTICE AND COMPRESS: Crushed fresh leaves can be applied as a poultice directly to bites or minor skin irritations. A cool compress can be used to reduce redness, swelling, and minor irritation from insect bites. A warm compress can be used on the temples or neck to ease tension headaches.

⚠ General Safety:

TOPICAL USE: Safe for most, but basil essential oil is very concentrated and can irritate sensitive skin.

INTERNAL USE: Safe in culinary recipes and tea. Strong tinctures should be used with care in those on blood-thinning medications. Culinary use is generally safe for pregnant and nursing women, but medicinal extracts in high amounts should be avoided without professional guidance.

HERBALIST TIP:

Basil leaves lose their flavor quickly when dried. For long-term storage, make pesto, freeze chopped leaves in olive oil, or dry them gently in very low heat to preserve more aroma and taste.

Blue Butterfly Pea Flower

Clitoria ternatea
Perennial in zones 9–12

This heat-loving, vining legume with striking deep blue (sometimes purple or white) blossoms is prized for its vivid natural dye, calming tea, and fun color-changing properties in drinks.

Medicinal Properties:

TOPICAL: A skin-soothing antioxidant; supports skin elasticity.

INTERNAL: A mild nervine that promotes cognitive support.

ENERGETIC: Cooling, slightly moistening.

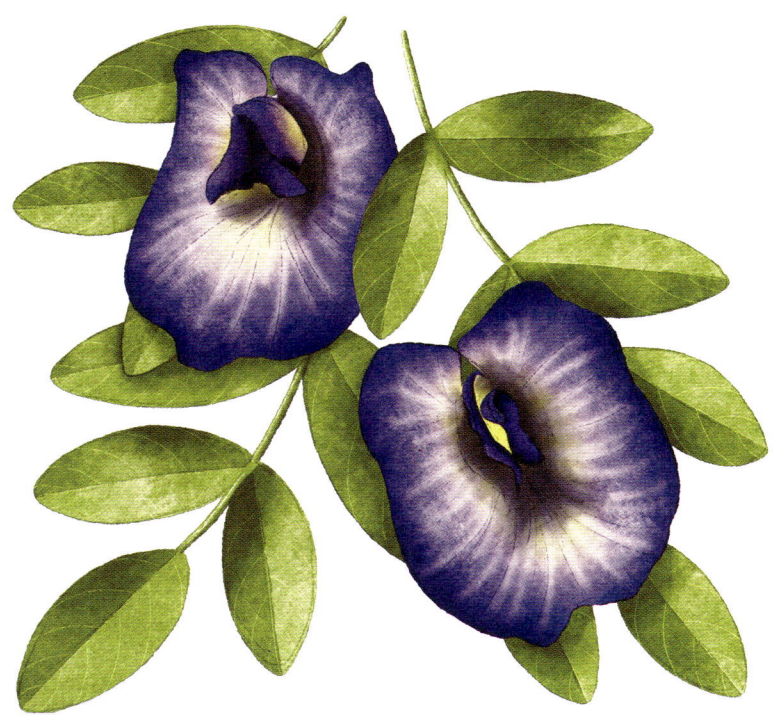

How to Grow:

 WHEN TO PLANT: Direct sow or transplant outdoors once soil temps are consistently above 60°F. This is always in early summer, after the threat of last frost has passed and nights have warmed a bit. Plants won't take off until warmer days arrive.

 GROWS BEST FROM: Seed or transplant. Nick the seeds, then soak them for 12–24 hours before planting. Germination can take 1–2 weeks. Using a heat mat for seeds started inside or in a grow room can be very helpful with germination. This herb transplants well and is often grown by home growers to be sold or traded locally.

 SUN AND SOIL NEEDS: Full sun, 6–8 hours or more, but tolerates partial shade. Likes well-draining, moderately fertile soil. Water regularly in early stages of growth. Can tolerate some drought once established.

 VARIETIES TO TRY: Single blue flower, double blue flower, and pink or white flower.

 SPACING: Space plants 18–24" apart. This is an aggressive vining plant! One healthy plant can cover almost 20' of trellis over a long, hot summer. You can plant a few in a large area, but more than one plant is typically not necessary in an average garden.

 BLOOM TIME: Flowers can appear in 60–90 days from seed, depending on how warm your soil temps and environment are at the time of planting.

 HARVESTING TIPS: Harvest flowers when they are fully open but still fresh. The best time to harvest is usually early in the day after morning dew has dried. Harvest daily or every other day during peak blooming, as the plant will continue producing blossoms (as long as you keep harvesting) until frost arrives.

GOOD TO KNOW:

Tea made with blue butterfly pea flowers changes color depending on the pH of the liquid the tea is made with or mixed with. The tea turns blue on its own, and purple/violet with the addition of lemon juice. This makes it a fun ingredient in tea blends thanks to its visual appeal.

How to Use:

 INFUSED OIL: Dried petals can be infused with skin-safe oils for a skin tonic.

 TINCTURE: Not typically tinctured for medicinal use.

 TEA: Steep 1 tablespoon dried flowers, or 5–6 fresh flowers, per 1 cup hot water for 5–10 minutes for reducing mental stress, increasing cognitive support, and extracting anthocyanins (beneficial pigments in plants like blueberries).

 POULTICE AND COMPRESS: Crushed fresh petals can be applied as a poultice for minor inflammation, or a cooling compress can be made with this herb for sunburns, heat rash, or puffy eyes.

⚠ General Safety:

TOPICAL USE: Well tolerated by most people, but those with sensitive skin may have irritation, redness, or burning with use. Avoid use on broken skin or open wounds.

INTERNAL USE: Generally safe in culinary and tea amounts for most adults and children. Considered safe in small tea/food amounts for pregnant or nursing mothers.

HERBALIST TIP:

Butterfly pea is a great herb to mix with other herbs that have opposing energetic qualities, like ginger, which is warming and drying, to help balance out a blend with its cooling and moistening energetics.

Blue Vervain

Verbena hastata
Perennial in zones 3–8

Blue vervain is a tall, slender perennial with striking spikes of tiny violet-blue flowers. Known as a nervine bitter, it has a long history of use in North American and European herbal traditions for supporting the liver and easing stress-related conditions.

Medicinal Properties:

TOPICAL: Used less often externally, but can be made into compresses or poultices for bruises, insect bites, or skin inflammation.

INTERNAL: Nervine relaxant that can help relieve anxiety, support low mood, and ease mild depression. Also an antispasmodic, emmenagogue, and bitter tonic.

ENERGETIC: Cooling, drying.

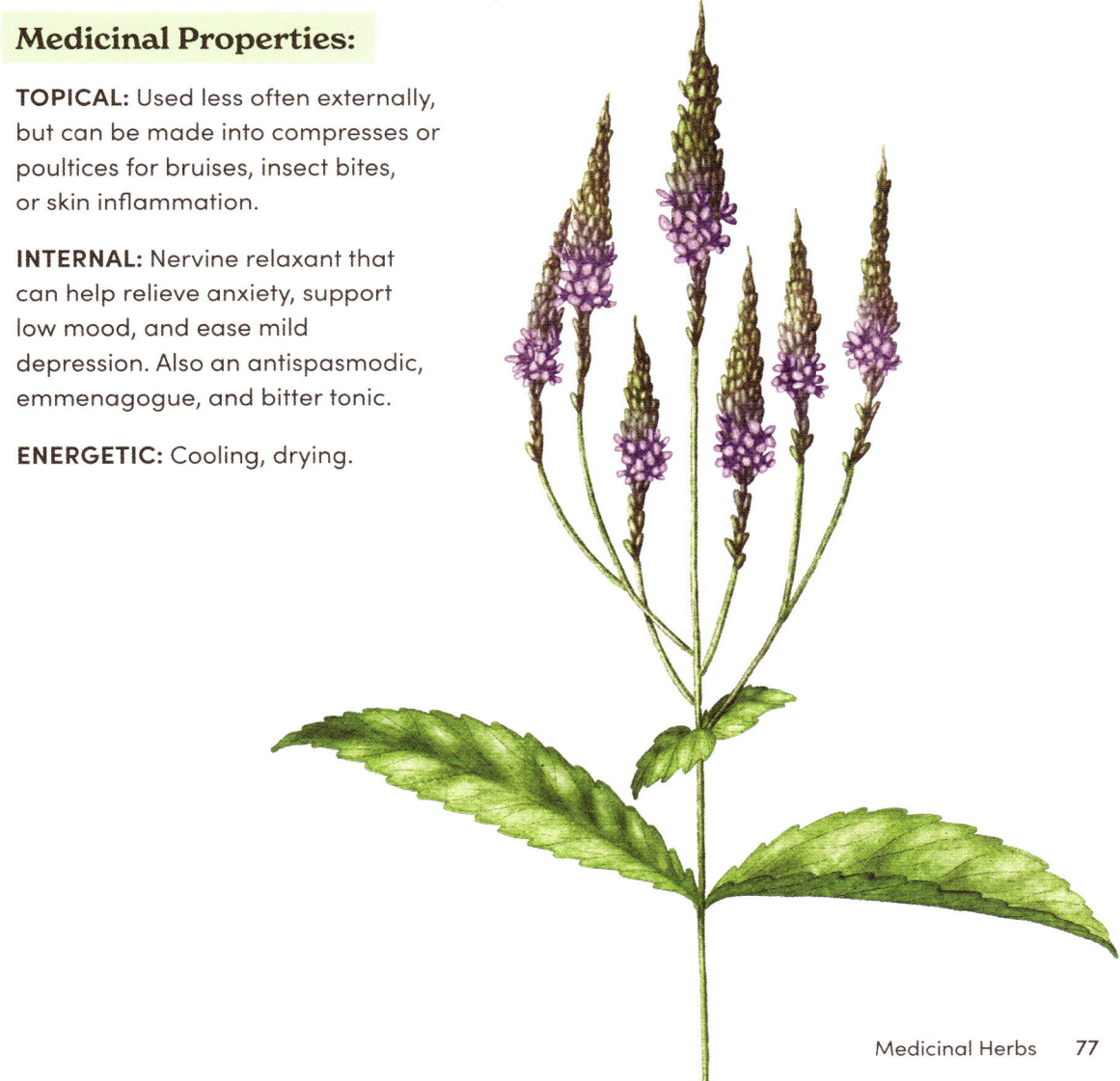

How to Grow:

 WHEN TO PLANT: Sow seeds outdoors in fall in mild winter climates, or in early spring in colder climates. Start indoors with a 4–6-week period of cold stratification. Transplant outdoors after the danger of frost has passed and when seedlings have at least 2–3 sets of true leaves.

 GROWS BEST FROM: Transplant, but can be started from seeds. Purchasing transplants of this herb is a best practice, as germination of seeds can be spotty and difficult. For cost-effectiveness when establishing a larger patch of this herb, consider starting from seed. Blue vervain seeds need to be cold stratified to achieve good germination indoors, or direct sown outside before winter to get the same effect.

 SUN AND SOIL NEEDS: Full sun to partial shade is best. In hotter regions, some afternoon shade is helpful to support the plant. Blue vervain prefers soil that stays consistently moist, much like the stream banks and meadows where it grows wild.

 VARIETIES TO TRY: Blue vervain and common vervain.

 SPACING: Space plants 12–18" apart. Blue vervain can reach 3–5' tall. Individual plants usually form clumps 1–2' wide at the base. Since it's a perennial with creeping roots, over time a single plant can expand into small colonies.

 BLOOM TIME: If you start this plant early indoors, you may see the summer blooms in the first year of growth, but the main flowering usually begins in the second year.

 HARVESTING TIPS: Aerial parts (flowers, stems, and leaves) should be harvested when the plant is in full flower for maximum potency. Cut the top 6–8" of the plant, including flowers and upper leaves. Leave some stalks behind so the plant can continue growing and self-seeding.

GOOD TO KNOW:

Blue vervain is considered stronger than many other nervines and is best suited for tense, overworked, type A personalities with chronic stress. It tastes extremely bitter, so tincture is often the preferred preparation over tea.

How to Use:

 INFUSED OIL: Not typically used infused into fat-based solvents. (Alcohol or water are better for extracting this herb's constituents.)

 TINCTURE: 1 part fresh herb to 2 parts 65–70% alcohol, or 1 part dried herb to 5 parts 40–50% alcohol to encourage deeper relaxation without heavy sedation, and as a mild antidepressant for those with nervous strain and exhaustion.

 TEA: Steep 1 teaspoon dried herb per 1 cup hot water for 10–15 minutes. Fresh herb is more bitter than dried, so is not typically suggested for tea preparations. Even dried blue vervain is very bitter and often blended with milder herbs like chamomile or mint. Used for calming an overactive mind at nighttime. In addition, the bitter notes can help aid in bile flow and liver function to support sluggish digestion.

 POULTICE AND COMPRESS: Crushed fresh leaves can be applied as a poultice to bruises or swollen areas. A warm or cool compress can be used to ease tension in the shoulders, neck, or jaw and to relieve tension headaches on temples.

 BATH SOAK: Dried aerial parts can be added to relaxing herbal bath blends for stress relief. Fresh leaves can also be used, but require a much higher volume, which makes this a less manageable option.

General Safety:

TOPICAL USE: Generally safe, though not often used externally.

INTERNAL USE: Avoid in high doses, as this herb may cause nausea due to strong bitterness. Blue vervain is not recommended during pregnancy, as it may stimulate uterine contractions. Nursing mothers should also avoid unless approved by a healthcare provider.

HERBALIST TIP:

Blue vervain works best for those who are tense, irritable, and mentally overactive. When stress shows up as neck/shoulder tightness, tension headaches, or insomnia, a few drops of tincture often go further than a cup of tea.

Calendula

Calendula officinalis
Annual

A cool season, low-growing, and flowering herb that can self-seed, calendula is best known for its vibrant orange and yellow flowers and its sticky resin.

Medicinal Properties:

TOPICAL: Wound healing; speeds tissue repair in cuts, scrapes, burns, insect bites, and rashes. It's also antibacterial and antifungal, so it helps prevent infection in minor wounds.

INTERNAL: Can soothe symptoms of sore throats, gastritis, ulcers, or intestinal inflammation. Stimulates lymphatic movement. High in antioxidants, so it can reduce inflammation.

ENERGETIC: Mildly warming, drying.

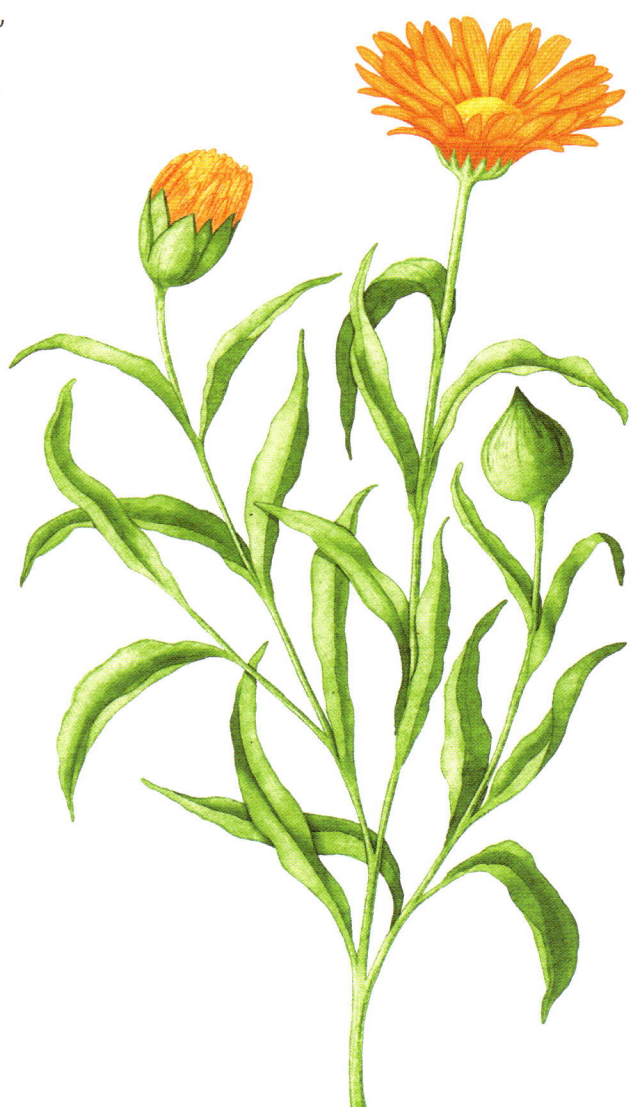

How to Grow:

 WHEN TO PLANT: In mild winter climates, it can be sown or transplanted in early fall. In northern gardens, sow after your last frost has passed in spring.

 GROWS BEST FROM: Seed or transplant. Plant seeds ¼" deep. Lightly cover with soil or compost and keep moist, but not waterlogged. Seeds benefit from darkness. Expect germination in 5–10 days.

 SUN AND SOIL NEEDS: Full sun, 6–8 hours or more, but afternoon shade is preferred in hotter months. Prefers moist soil.

 VARIETIES TO TRY: Resina, Oopsy Daisy, Pacific Beauty, Oktoberfest, Orange King, Pink Surprise, and Geisha Girl.

 SPACING: Space plants 18–24" apart. Allowing for adequate spacing in between plants can help avoid fungal issues due to poor airflow and increase the energy available to produce more flowers. Container friendly.

 BLOOM TIME: 50–70 days after transplanting. Add 2–3 weeks to this timeline if direct sowing.

 HARVESTING TIPS: Harvesting begins once buds are half open to fully open. Harvest flower heads early in the day, after dew dries but before full sun exposure. Pick when petals are open and vibrant, but before they begin to wilt or fade. To enccurage continuous blooming, deadhead (remove spent blooms) and harvest fresh blooms regularly.

GROWING TIP:

Calendula is a beautiful flower, but it can be sticky! It's known to smell quite "medicinal," and harvesting it can coat your hands with a sticky sap. This sap is referred to as the "resin" of the plant, and it contains the majority of its medicinal properties. Pollinators will visit these blooms, but calendula is not the top pollinator magnet in a fully blooming spring garden.

How to Use:

 INFUSED OIL: For skin conditions, dried or freshly wilted calendula petals can be infused into salves, oils, and diaper rash creams.

 TINCTURE: 1 part fresh flowers to 2 parts 50–60% alcohol. Fresh flowers are best for the use of resins. Used as a strong lymphagogue to help stimulate lymphatic flow and reduce inflammation in tissues and clear waste and to soothe inflamed mucous membranes in the stomach, intestines, or throat.

 TEA: Steep 2–3 teaspoons dried petals, or 2–3 tablespoons fresh petals, per 1 cup hot water, covered, for 10–15 minutes. Best blended with supporting herbs. Gentle and soothing to the stomach and throat.

 POULTICE AND COMPRESS: Crushed fresh petals and leaves can be applied as a poultice to wounds to speed healing. A warm or cool compress can be used to treat fungal skin irritations and minor cuts, scrapes, and burns, or as an eye compress for conjunctivitis.

⚠ General Safety:

TOPICAL USE: Very well tolerated by most people. Those allergic to plants in the Asteraceae (daisy) family may have mild skin rashes and reactions.

INTERNAL USE: Not recommended for pregnant or nursing mothers. Avoid if currently prescribed a sedative, antihypertensive, or central nervous system (CNS) depressant.

HERBALIST TIP:

To maximize potency in your calendula preparations:

❀ Harvest flowers in the heat of the day, when resins are strongest.
❀ Use whole flower heads in oil infusions or tinctures, not just petals.
❀ Consider slightly wilting fresh flowers before infusing in oil to reduce water content but retain resins.

California Poppy

Eschscholzia californica

Short-lived perennial in zones 6–10

This low-growing herb has feathery, blue-green foliage and bright orange to golden cup-shaped flowers.

Medicinal Properties:

TOPICAL: Not commonly used externally.

INTERNAL: Mild sedative, nervine that eases insomnia, analgesic, and antispasmodic that can ease menstrual cramps and muscle soreness.

ENERGETIC: Cooling, drying.

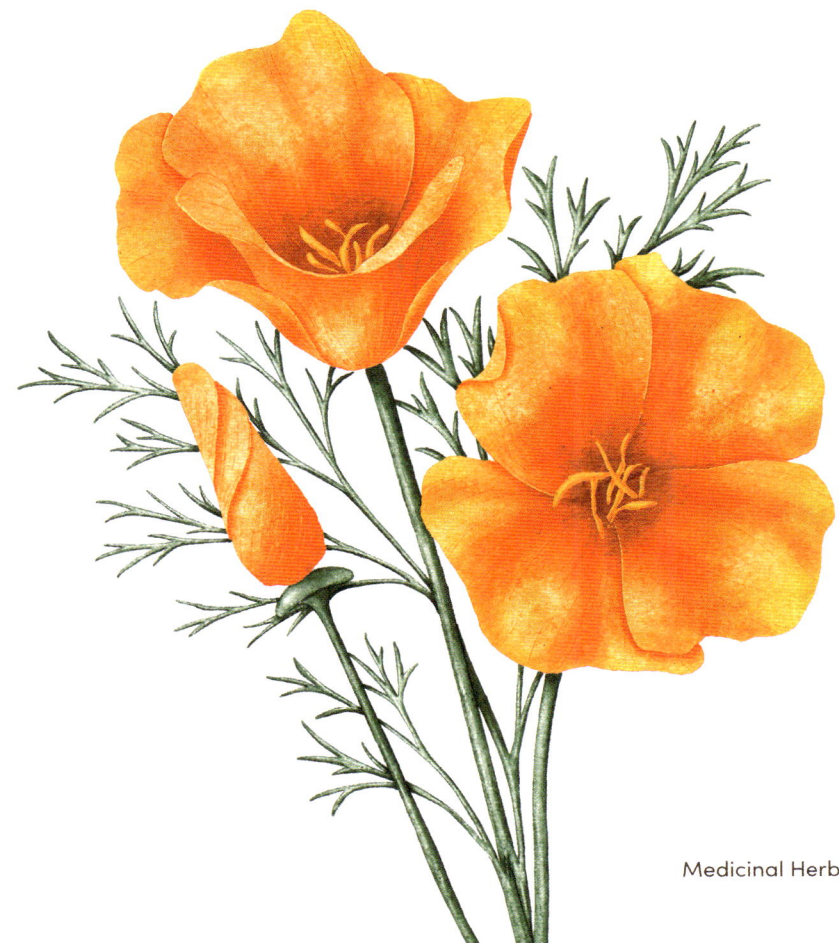

How to Grow:

 WHEN TO PLANT: Direct sow outdoors in fall in warmer winter regions as a wildflower, or in early spring in colder winter regions.

 GROWS BEST FROM: Seed; does not transplant well. Direct sowing is strongly preferred. This herb, like other poppies, benefits from cold stratification to mimic outdoor wild growing conditions.

 SUN AND SOIL NEEDS: Full sun, 6–8 hours or more, for best blooms. Prefers sandy or rocky soil with good drainage. Drought tolerant once established.

 VARIETIES TO TRY: Mikado, Mission Bells, and Classic Orange.

 SPACING: Sow seeds 6–8" apart for compact growth. California poppy grows in patches and can reseed to spread into larger areas. Plants can get 12–18" tall.

 BLOOM TIME: Aerial tops are ready for harvest in 55–70 days after sowing.

 HARVESTING TIPS: Peak harvest is midsummer, when plants are in full flower.

GOOD TO KNOW:

California poppy is the official state flower of California and was widely used by Indigenous people of the West Coast for calming restlessness, easing toothaches, and promoting sleep. Unlike the opium poppy, California poppy is nonaddictive and safe in moderate use.

How to Use:

 INFUSED OIL: Not typically made with this herb.

 TINCTURE: 1 part fresh aerial parts to 2 parts 50–60% alcohol, or 1 part dried herb to 5 parts 40–50% alcohol. Used for anxiety, restlessness, and mild insomnia.

 TEA: Steep 1 tablespoon dried aerial parts, or ¼ cup fresh packed aerial parts, per 1 cup hot water for 10–15 minutes. Dried California poppies are more bitter than fresh, but are better suited for adults with moderate anxiety, insomnia, or muscle tension. Fresh herbs are better suited for children and gentle nervine use.

 POULTICE AND COMPRESS: A poultice is not typically made with this herb. A warm compress can help relieve tension in the body.

 SYRUP: Prepared for children as a gentle sleep aid.

 General Safety:

TOPICAL USE: Rarely used externally.

INTERNAL USE: Safe in moderate doses. May cause mild drowsiness. Can enhance sedatives or sleep medications, so avoid combining without guidance. Avoid strong medicinal doses if pregnant or nursing, as limited safety data is available.

HERBALIST TIP:

California poppy is one of the best gentle nervines for children and sensitive individuals, especially when blended with lemon balm, chamomile, or passion vine for sleep and relaxation.

Catnip

Nepeta cataria

Perennial in zones 3–9 (variety dependent)

This gray-green, fuzzy-leafed herb with spikes of white to pink or lavender flowers is famous for its effect on cats, but it is also a valuable medicinal and pollinator-friendly plant for humans.

Medicinal Properties:

TOPICAL: Relieves mild skin irritation and itching. Can be used as a natural insect repellent.

INTERNAL: Carminative that relieves gas, bloating, indigestion, and colic in infants. Nervine that eases anxiety and stress; mild sedative. Helps ease coughs and congestion. Mild diaphoretic.

ENERGETIC: Cooling, drying.

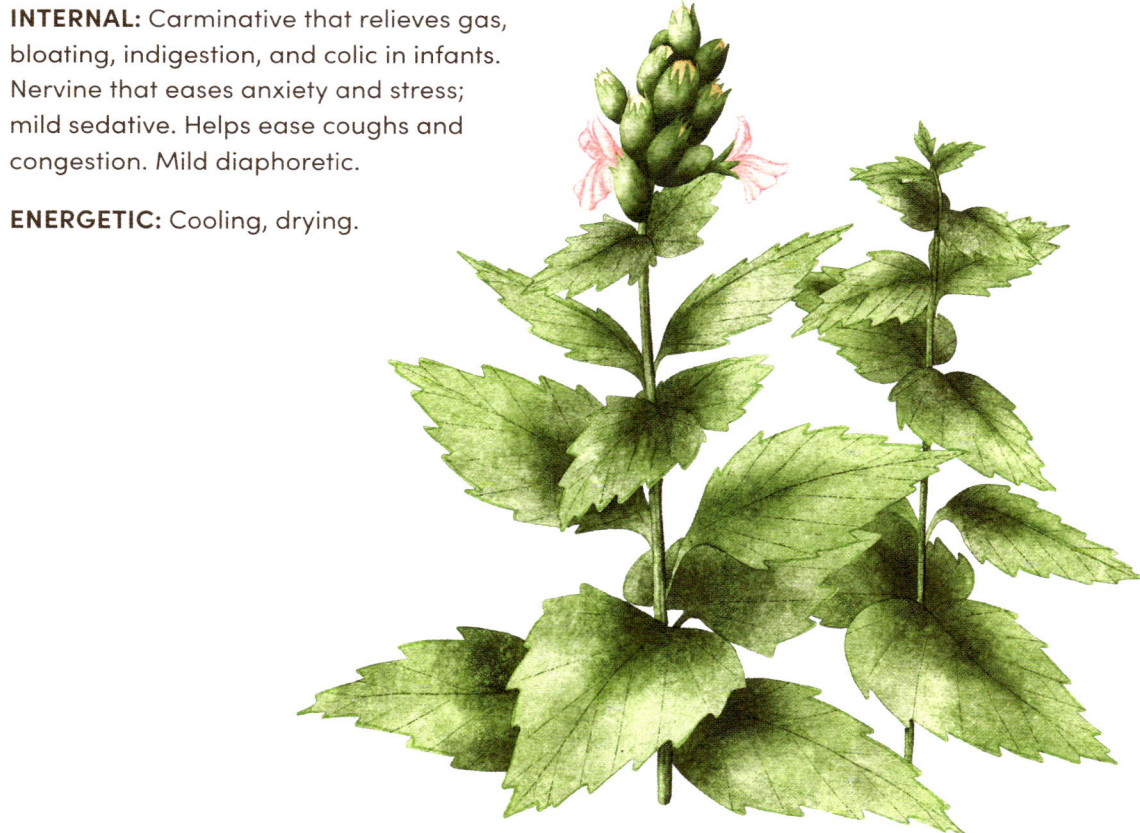

How to Grow:

 WHEN TO PLANT: Sow or transplant after the danger of frost has passed. In mild climates, start seeds indoors 6–8 weeks before last frost.

 GROWS BEST FROM: Seed, transplant, or propagation. Sow seeds on the soil surface and gently press in. Keep soil moist and warm for better germination. Seeds need light to germinate. Germination can take 7–14 days. Direct sowing may be difficult with how tiny the seeds are. Catnip easily propagates in water or soil. Divide established clumps in spring or fall.

 SUN AND SOIL NEEDS: Full sun to partial shade. More shade in hotter climates, specifically in the afternoon. Prefers slightly sandy, well-draining soil with moderate, consistent moisture. More sun will produce catnip with stronger fragrance and potency.

 VARIETIES TO TRY: Common catnip, Greek catnip, lemon catnip, and ornamental nepeta (for pollinators).

 SPACING: Space plants 18–24" apart for vigorous spread. Catnip will quickly fill in gaps, so this spacing gives each plant room to breathe without overcrowding. In containers, space one plant per 12–16"-diameter pot for full, bushy growth. Use a deep pot (at least 10–12") to keep roots contained. Place a self-watering dish or base under pots to help avoid the spread of runners via catnip's rhizomatous root system.

 BLOOM TIME: 60–90 days from seed to initial small harvest. 90–100 days from seed to a time when plants are well established. Produces flowers in the summer.

 HARVESTING TIPS: Begin harvesting leaves once plants are at least 8–12" tall. The best flavor and potency is just before plants start to flower. If you need usable leaves sooner, start catnip from cuttings or divisions. You can harvest within 4–6 weeks instead of waiting 2–3 months from seed.

GOOD TO KNOW:

Cats typically prefer the dried herb over the fresh, as the nepetalactone (the active compound) intensifies as the plant dries.

How to Use:

 INFUSED OIL: Dried leaves can be infused into oils, salves, and balms for topical use. Catnip is helpful in natural insect-repelling balms.

 TINCTURE: 1 part fresh herb to 2 parts 40% alcohol, or 1 part dried herb to 5 parts 50–60% alcohol. Tincture when fresh to preserve the volatile oils. Use as a concentrated nervine support and useful sleep aid.

 TEA: Steep 1 tablespoon dried leaves, or ¼ cup fresh leaves, covered, per 1 cup hot water or cold water for 10–15 minutes. Used as a gentle nervine to ease stress and anxiety and to relieve mild bloating, flatulence, and indigestion. Also used to help break a fever as a diaphoretic.

 POULTICE AND COMPRESS: Used in poultices to help with headaches (apply to temples), mild skin irritation, and bug bites. Compresses have similar use and also aid in fever support.

〰️ **STEAM INHALATION:** Add a handful of fresh leaves, or 1 tablespoon dried leaves, to a bowl of hot water. Tent your head with a towel and inhale vapors for 5–10 minutes to loosen mucous and open nasal passages.

⚠️ General Safety:

TOPICAL USE: Well tolerated by most people, but volatile oils can irritate sensitive skin. Always patch test for safety.

INTERNAL USE: Generally safe in culinary and tea amounts for most adults and children. Traditionally avoided in large medicinal doses during pregnancy due to its mild uterine-stimulating effects.

HERBALIST TIP:

Catnip is known for spreading very aggressively in the garden. It also has a very "dank" smell. So consider planting it in containers, or you risk having it take over your space!

Chamomile

Matricaria recutita syn. Matricaria chamomilla
Annual

A gentle, daisy-like herb with feathery foliage and small white and yellow flowers, chamomile has long been valued as a calming remedy and soothing digestive aid.

Medicinal Properties:

TOPICAL: Soothes eczema, rashes, burns, wounds, insect bites, stings, or inflamed skin.

INTERNAL: Antispasmodic. Calms nervous tension and supports low mood/depression, irritability, and insomnia. Eases gas colic, indigestion, and nausea. Helpful for children with teething, fussiness, upset stomachs, and sore throats.

ENERGETIC: Cooling, drying.

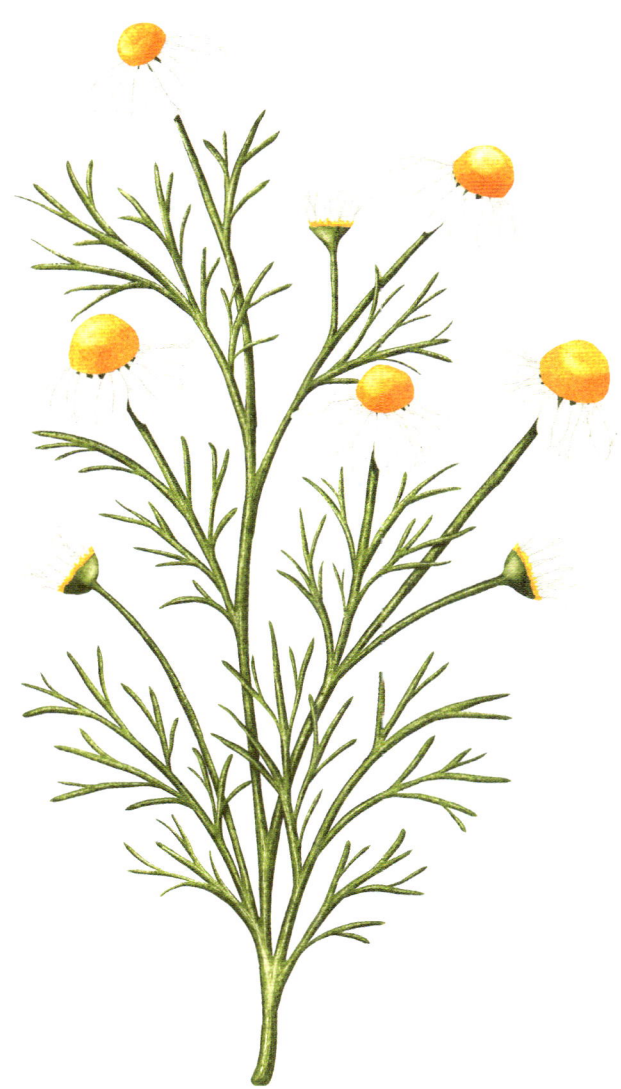

How to Grow:

 WHEN TO PLANT: Direct sow into the garden as soon as soil can be worked. You can sow chamomile before the last frost in mild climates, and it will come up and bloom with the first flowers of the growing season. It can also be transplanted and covered lightly during hard frosts below 25°F in mild winter climates to help get a head start on the growing season in early spring.

 GROWS BEST FROM: Seed or transplant. The seeds are very small and should be sowed on the surface of the soil and kept moist with a spray bottle of water. Germination is quick and can happen in as little as 5–10 days. Sow seed densely, as chamomile does fine bunched up together. Transplant anytime between fall and late February in warmer regions. Wait until the last frost has passed in cooler regions.

 SUN AND SOIL NEEDS: Full sun, 6–8 hours or more, for best blooms. In hotter regions, be sure to harvest regularly to keep blooms and plants fresh and thriving. Does best with well-draining soil, but needs regular moisture to thrive.

 VARIETIES TO TRY: German chamomile and Roman chamomile.

 SPACING: Space plants 8–12" apart. Plants are small and airy, so they don't need wide spacing, but they do benefit from airflow to reduce mildew. You can plant more densely if you want them to act more like a ground cover, but they will get taller once blooms shoot up.

 BLOOM TIME: 60–70 days from seed to initial small harvest during active growing season. When sown in the fall/winter in mild climates, blooms will appear in early spring.

 HARVESTING TIPS: Harvest blooms as soon as they open, and harvest them daily. This will encourage more blooms and allow peak production.

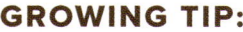

GROWING TIP:

Although it is an annual, chamomile can reseed effectively on its own, so a smaller chamomile patch can come back bigger each year if you let some blooms go to seed.

How to Use:

 INFUSED OIL: Dried or freshly wilted flowers can be infused into oils, salves, and balms for skin-calming treatments.

 TINCTURE: 1 part fresh aerial parts to 2 parts 50% alcohol, or 1 part dried aerial parts to 5 parts 40% alcohol. Used for reducing stress and anxiety, promoting restful sleep, and calming nightmares. Chamomile can also be used as an antispasmodic to help relax the smooth muscles of the digestive tract to reduce stomach cramps, gas, bloating, and menstrual cramps.

 TEA: Steep 1 tablespoon dried flowers, or 2–3 tablespoons fresh flowers, covered, per 1 cup hot water, for 10–15 minutes to soothe nausea, anxiety, sore throats, and trapped gas, and to support restful sleep.

 POULTICE AND COMPRESS: Used in poultices to soothe inflamed areas and in warm compresses on the abdomen to help reduce menstrual cramps.

 BATH SOAK: Add chamomile flowers to a warm bath for full-body relaxation.

General Safety:

TOPICAL USE: Well tolerated by most people. Those with allergies to plants in the ragweed family should avoid chamomile.

INTERNAL USE: Generclly safe in culinary and tea amounts for most children and adults, including pregnant and nursing women. Strong preparations should be used with caution alongside blood-thinning medications.

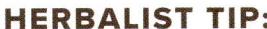

HERBALIST TIP:

Chamomile has an apple-like aroma, and even though the tea is mild in flavor, it is an effective nervine and digestive aid that can help with menstrual cramp pain as well. Chamomile tea works best for cramps when started a few days before menstruation begins, as it keeps inflammation and muscle tension from building up.

Cilantro

Coriandrum sativum
Annual

Cilantro is a fast-growing, leafy herb with delicate, lacy green foliage and a strong, distinct flavor. Both the fresh leaves and the dried seeds are widely used in culinary and medicinal traditions around the world.

Medicinal Properties:

TOPICAL: Skin soothing, cooling, antimicrobial.

INTERNAL: Antifungal. Detoxes heavy metals. Supports digestion and reduces gas and bloat.

ENERGETIC: Cooling, moistening.

GROWING TIP:

Cilantro bolts in hot weather, sending up tall flower stalks and forming seeds that are referred to as coriander. In some countries, the leafy portion of the cilantro plant is also referred to as coriander, which can be confusing! Resowing cilantro every 2–3 weeks in cooler weather can help you maintain a steady supply of fresh leaves. The bolted cilantro plant is a great host plant for ladybugs, so let some of your plants go to seed to help bring beneficial insects into the garden.

How to Grow:

 WHEN TO PLANT: In milder climates, direct sow seeds starting in fall throughout the winter. Cilantro prefers cooler temperatures and can tolerate light frosts. In colder regions, direct sow after the last frost has passed in spring.

 GROWS BEST FROM: Seed; does not transplant well. Seeds germinate in 7–14 days. The coriander seed (cilantro seed) is actually two seeds in one, so cracking open the seeds with a rolling pin and soaking them for 1 day in water will aid in germination. Sprinkle seeds liberally across the soil surface and lightly cover with soil to keep moist. Moisture is key for good germination within the first 2 weeks.

 SUN AND SOIL NEEDS: Full sun to partial shade. In hotter summer climates, some afternoon shade can help your cilantro stay tastier longer (instead of wilting or bolting and going to seed). Prefers consistent moisture in well-draining soil amended well with organic matter. Grows very well in containers.

 VARIETIES TO TRY: Slo-Bolt, Santo, Calypso, Cruiser, Caribe, Moroccan coriander, Leisure, and Delfino.

 SPACING: Sow seeds 2–3" apart in rows or scatter sow and thin to 4–6" apart. Plants don't mind growing fairly close if harvested young for leaves. Full-sized plants for leaf and seed can benefit from being spaced 8–10" apart in rows that are 12–15" apart. This allows airflow and reduces bolting stress, specifically in warmer southern regions.

 BLOOM TIME: Typically 30–40 days from seed to leaf harvest and 90–100 days for cilantro to reach the flowering and "going to seed" stage (coriander).

 HARVESTING TIPS: Cut outer leaves first or harvest whole plants at once. For seeds, allow plants to flower, and dry seed heads on the stalk before collecting.

How to Use:

 INFUSED OIL: Fresh cilantro leaves are not ideal for oil infusion due to their high water content, but coriander seeds can be infused to make digestive oils or salves. Both oils and salves can be rubbed onto the abdomen externally for digestive relief.

 TINCTURE: Not typically tinctured for medicinal use.

 TEA: Steep 1–2 teaspoons crushed coriander seeds per 1 cup hot water for 10–15 minutes to aid digestion. (Fresh leaves are less commonly used for tea.)

 POULTICE AND COMPRESS: Crushed fresh leaves can be applied as a poultice directly to the skin for itching, irritation, or mild rashes. A cool compress can be made to help soothe bug bite irritation, inflammation, and puffy eyes.

 General Safety:

TOPICAL USE: Generally safe, but may rarely cause skin sensitivity in some individuals.

INTERNAL USE: Safe in culinary and medicinal amounts. Seeds are gentler on digestion than leaves for sensitive stomachs. Considered safe in food amounts for pregnant and nursing women, but medicinal doses should be used with caution, especially seed extracts.

HERBALIST TIP:

Cilantro seed (coriander) combines beautifully with digestive herbs, like fennel and mint, to make a light after-meal tea or fresh garnish blend that relieves bloating and freshens breath. You can also put cilantro leaves in fresh salsa, salads, and broths, or blend it into juices with other vegetables and fruits for blood-detoxifying properties.

Comfrey

Symphytum officinale
Winter hardy perennial in zones 3–9

This cool season, fast-growing understory perennial has large, fuzzy leaves and nodding purple, blue, or pink bell-shaped flowers. It is traditionally used for rapid wound and bone healing, which has earned it the nickname "knitbone."

Medicinal Properties:

TOPICAL: Can speed tissue and bone repair and soothe sprains, bruises, strains, and inflammation. Known to help regenerate skin cells and reduce burst blood vessels. Helpful for reducing bruising at a quicker rate than without application.

INTERNAL: Not used internally.

ENERGETIC: Cooling, moistening.

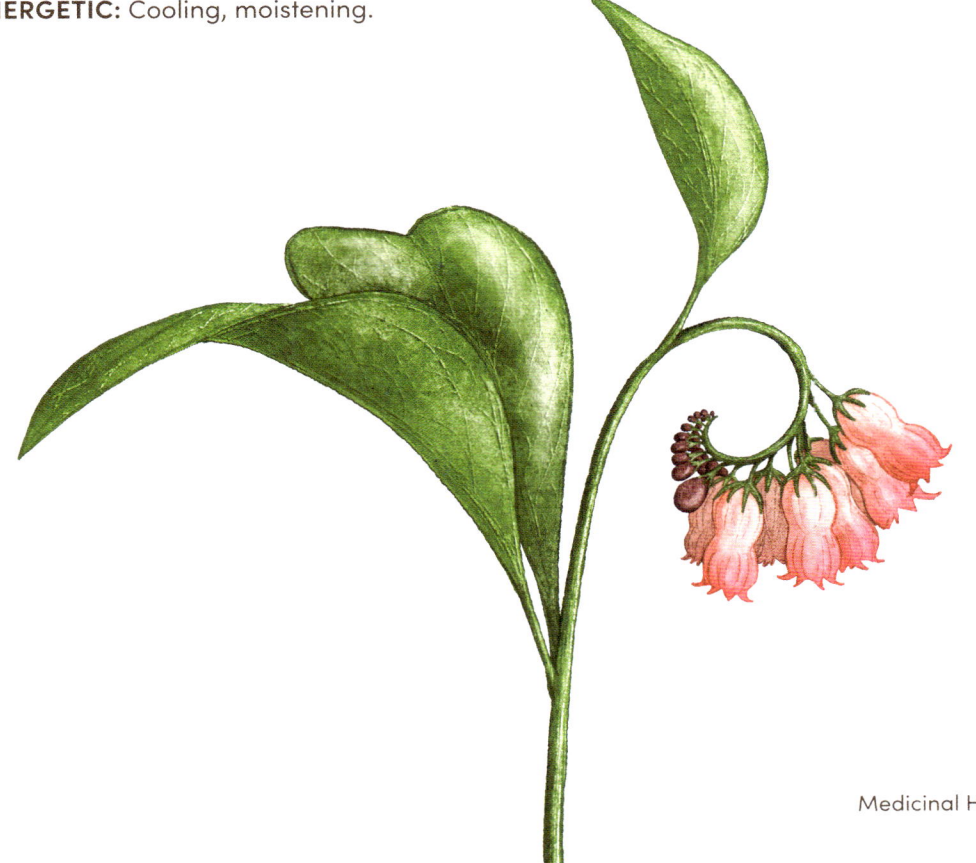

How to Grow:

 WHEN TO PLANT: Can be transplanted in early fall in mild winter climates. In northern gardens, sow or transplant after the last frost has passed in spring.

 GROWS BEST FROM: Seed for true comfrey varieties and root division for sterile varieties.

 SUN AND SOIL NEEDS: Full sun to partial shade. Thrives in moist, fertile soil.

 VARIETIES TO TRY: Russian Bocking 14 and true comfrey.

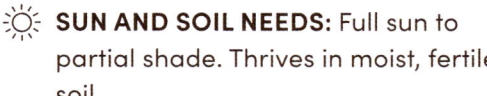 **SPACING:** Space plants 24–36" apart—plants can get quite large.

 BLOOM TIME: True comfrey may establish and bloom within 6–12 months. The seeds need to be cold stratified for 4–6 weeks in moist conditions before planting. Germination can take anywhere from 2–6 weeks, and the seedling-to-plantable stage can take even longer. Although the seeds of the Russian Bocking 14 variety are sterile, the plant can bloom on its second season.

 HARVESTING TIPS: Harvest leaves before flowering for best potency. You should be able to take leaves from the plant 3 or 4 times per season without damaging its overall health as long as you leave a few leaves to regrow each time.

GROWING TIP:

Comfrey leaves are coarse and hairy, so wearing gloves during harvest can be helpful. True comfrey (*Symphytum officinale*) can be grown from seed, but it does drop seeds throughout the season—so plant it in an area that has room for it to spread. Russian Bocking 14 is a sterile, hybrid variety of comfrey that is lower in herbal properties but is preferred for smaller gardens because it stays where it's planted.

How to Use:

 INFUSED OIL: Can be dried and infused into skin-safe oils to apply to sprains, sore joints, bruises, and wounds (but not open or deep puncture wounds), or mixed with beeswax for a muscle rub salve.

 TINCTURE: Not recommended for this herb.

 TEA: Not recommended for this herb.

 POULTICE AND COMPRESS: Crushed fresh leaves can be applied as a poultice to help heal tissue, reduce bruising, and reduce inflammation. For a compress, steep dried leaves in hot water, soak a cloth, and apply to sore areas for similar support.

General Safety:

TOPICAL USE: Safe for external use on closed wounds and unbroken skin. Comfrey can heal skin *so* fast that it may actually seal in infection if applied to dirty or deep wounds, so never apply to those areas.

INTERNAL USE: Not recommended, due to potential liver toxicity.

HERBALIST TIP:

Dehydrating comfrey leaves and grinding them into a powder can be a great way to keep comfrey on hand at all times, even in the winter. You can easily rehydrate this form of the herb to make a poultice, infusion, or compress.

Cornflower

Centaurea cyanus
Perennial in zones 3–9 (variety dependent)

Also known as bachelor's button, cornflower is a hardy annual with striking blue blossoms. Although traditionally grown as an ornamental or wildflower, it also has gentle medicinal uses and is valued for its beauty in pollinator gardens and herbal teas.

Medicinal Properties:

TOPICAL: Eye wash and soothing toner for scrapes and skin inflammation.

INTERNAL: Gentle digestive aid with mildly bitter properties. A cool tea calms fevers and mild inflammation.

ENERGETIC: Cooling, drying.

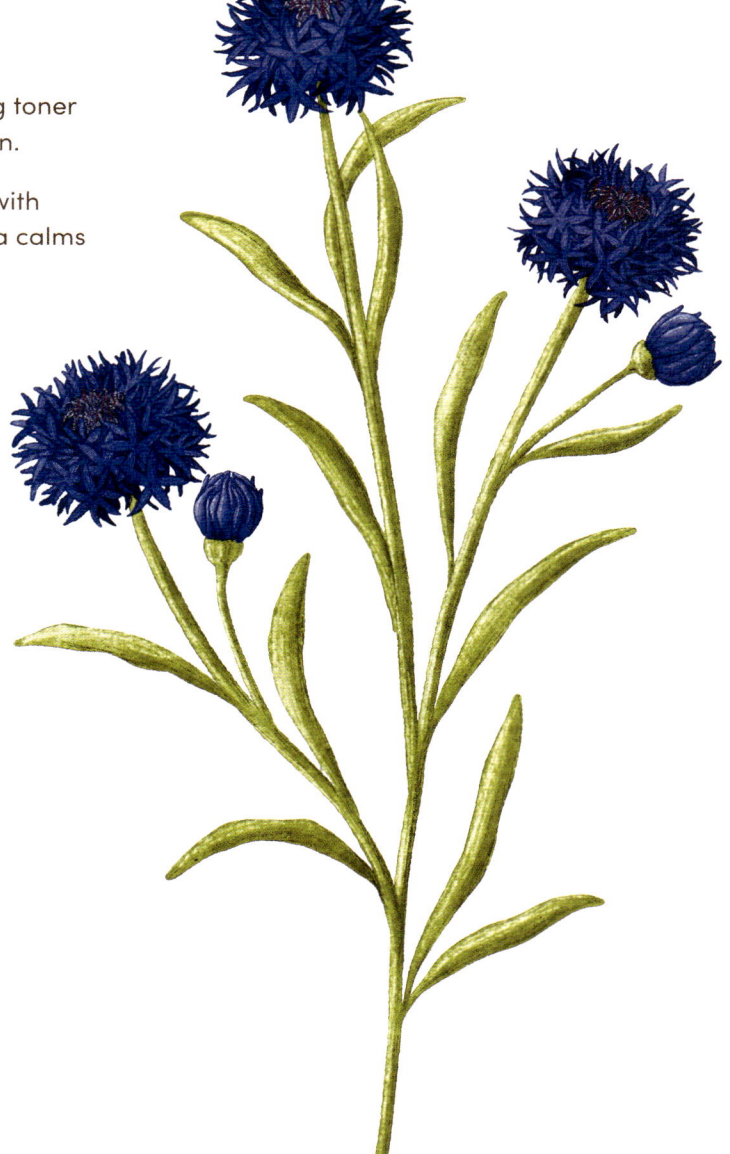

How to Grow:

 WHEN TO PLANT: Direct sow into the garden as soon as the soil can be worked. In mild climates, you can even sow cornflower before the last frost.

 GROWS BEST FROM: Seed; does not transplant well.

 SUN AND SOIL NEEDS: Full sun, 6–8 hours or more, for best blooms. In hotter regions, be sure to harvest regularly to keep blooms and plants fresh and thriving. Does best with loose, well-draining soil but tolerates poorer soils as long as the plants don't sit in wet, heavy ground.

 VARIETIES TO TRY: Classic blue cornflower, Black Ball, Polka Dot Mix, and Frosted Queen Mix.

 SPACING: Sow seeds or thin plants in place at 6–12" apart, depending on whether growing in rows or clusters. Plants get tall and floppy if not grown in patches.

 BLOOM TIME: 65–75 days from seed to initial small harvest during active growing season. When sown in the fall/winter in mild climates, blooms will appear in early spring.

 HARVESTING TIPS: Harvest blooms as soon as they open and harvest them daily. This will encourage more blooms and allow peak production from your cornflower plants.

GOOD TO KNOW:

Cornflowers are edible and often used in natural dye or as a garnish. Their vivid blue petals retain their color well when dried, making them popular in herbal tea blends for visual appeal.

How to Use:

 INFUSED OIL: Infuse dried petals into oils, salves, and balms for skin-calming treatments.

 TINCTURE: 1 part fresh herb to 2 parts 40–50% alcohol, or 1 part dried herb to 5 parts 40% alcohol. Supports urinary tract cleansing and sluggish digestion.

 TEA: Steep 1–2 teaspoons dried petals (usually blended with other herbs), covered, per 1 cup hot water for 10–15 minutes to help cool the body and support slow digestion. (Fresh petals are very mild in tea blends so it's best to use dried.)

 POULTICE AND COMPRESS: Used in poultices and compresses to help soothe eyes and skin irritation.

 General Safety:

TOPICAL USE: Well tolerated by most people. Those with allergies to plants in the Asteraceae (daisy) family should avoid cornflower.

INTERNAL USE: Generally safe in culinary and tea amounts for most adults and children.

HERBALIST TIP:

You can also make a facial toner out of cornflower. Simply steep a strong tea, strain, and cool completely. Store in the fridge and use under eyes and on face to reduce redness and puffiness.

Dandelion

Taraxacum officinale
Perennial in zones 3–10

Often thought of as a common weed, dandelion is actually a powerhouse of a medicinal herb. Its roots, leaves, and flowers are all useful, supporting the liver, kidneys, skin, and digestion while also offering nutritional value.

Medicinal Properties:

TOPICAL: Fresh flowers infused into oil are used for joint and muscle aches, sore breasts, and inflamed skin.

INTERNAL: Leaves are diuretic and rich in potassium, and they support kidney health and fluid balance. Roots are a bitter tonic that stimulates liver, bile flow, and digestion. Often used to support detoxification and skin health. Flowers are a mild antioxidant and mood lifter.

ENERGETIC: Cooling, drying.

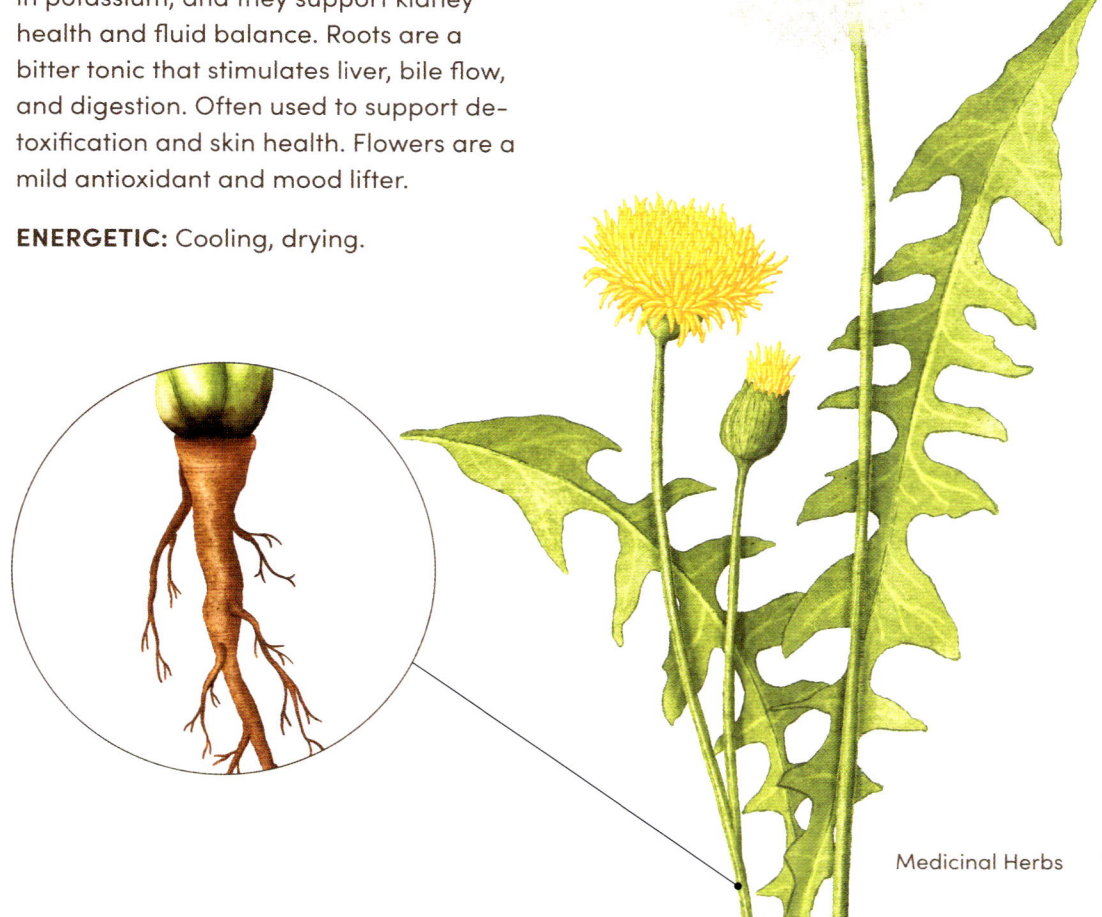

How to Grow:

 WHEN TO PLANT: Seeds can be sown directly outdoors in spring or fall.

 GROWS BEST FROM: Seed, though existing plants are often abundant in gardens and fields.

 SUN AND SOIL NEEDS: Full sun, 6–8 hours or more. Tolerates almost any soil, but prefers well-drained, moderately rich soil. Dandelions possess qualities that allow them to survive in less-than-ideal conditions.

 VARIETIES TO TRY: Common wild dandelion, Asian dandelion, and red-seeded dandelion.

 SPACING: If intentionally cultivating, space plants 6–12" apart. They will self-sow and spread naturally. Dandelions often naturally grow close together, but the more space you give each plant, the bigger the roots the plants can establish.

 BLOOM TIME: First flowers should appear about 8 weeks after sowing. Dandelions typically produce flowers for 8–15 weeks before going mostly to seed.

 HARVESTING TIPS: Ready to harvest 8 weeks after sowing or as soon as plants are established. Best picked young in spring for milder flavor. Roots are ready to harvest in the fall of the second year (18–24 months after sowing). This is when medicinal compounds are strongest. You can harvest a few leaves for teas or poultices in the first year, but the root should be left intact.

GOOD TO KNOW:

Young dandelion leaves are edible as a spring green, offering high levels of calcium, magnesium, iron, and potassium. Unlike many diuretics, dandelion leaves replace potassium lost through urination. Young leaves can also be juiced or used in salads for both flavor and medicinal benefit. The roots are best harvested in the fall of the second year. Dandelion flowers can be used to make wine, honey infusions, or skin salves.

How to Use:

 INFUSED OIL: Freshly wilted dandelion flowers can be infused for sore muscle relief, breast massage oil, or salves.

 TINCTURE: 1 part fresh root to 2 parts 65–70% alcohol, or 1 part dried root to 5 parts 40–50% alcohol, or 1 part fresh leaf to 2 parts 50–60% alcohol. Used as a digestive aid to increase bile flow and support the liver.

 TEA: Steep 1–2 teaspoons dried leaves per 1 cup hot water for 10–15 minutes (fresh leaves have a more grassy flavor that is less palatable, so use dried). You can also make a decoction by simmering 1 teaspoon dried chopped root in 1 cup water for 10–15 minutes. Do not simmer too long to avoid bitter flavors concentrating. Used for aiding in sluggish digestion, supporting the liver, and reducing inflammation and bloating.

 POULTICE AND COMPRESS: Crushed fresh leaves can be applied as a poultice to stings, bites, or inflamed skin. Cool compresses can be used to soothe sunburns, rashes, hives, eczema, and psoriasis flareups.

General Safety:

TOPICAL USE: Generally safe, but may cause mild skin irritation in rare cases.

INTERNAL USE: Safe in food and tea amounts. Large doses may cause digestive upset to sensitive stomachs. Generally considered safe in moderate amounts for pregnant and nursing women, but avoid strong medicinal doses without guidance.

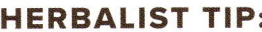

HERBALIST TIP:

Dandelion root combines beautifully with burdock root in decoctions for liver and skin health. Dandelion has year-round applications: Steep the leaves to make a gentle mineral-rich tea in spring, decoct the roots in autumn for deeper detoxification, and use flowers for uplifting remedies all year.

Echinacea

Echinacea purpurea, Echinacea angustifolia, Echinacea pallida
Short-lived perennial in zones 3–9

A hardy perennial with striking purple to pink coneflowers and spiny central cones, echinacea is a cornerstone of traditional herbal medicine because it supports the immune system and fights infection.

Medicinal Properties:

TOPICAL: Antiseptic and wound healing. Applied to cuts, insect bites, stings, and minor infections to reduce pain and swelling.

INTERNAL: Immunostimulant that can help the body resist colds, flu, and infections. Anti-inflammatory for sore throats and gum infections. Lymphagogue that can help with circulatory sluggishness and lymph stagnation along with urinary tract issues.

ENERGETIC: Cooling, drying.

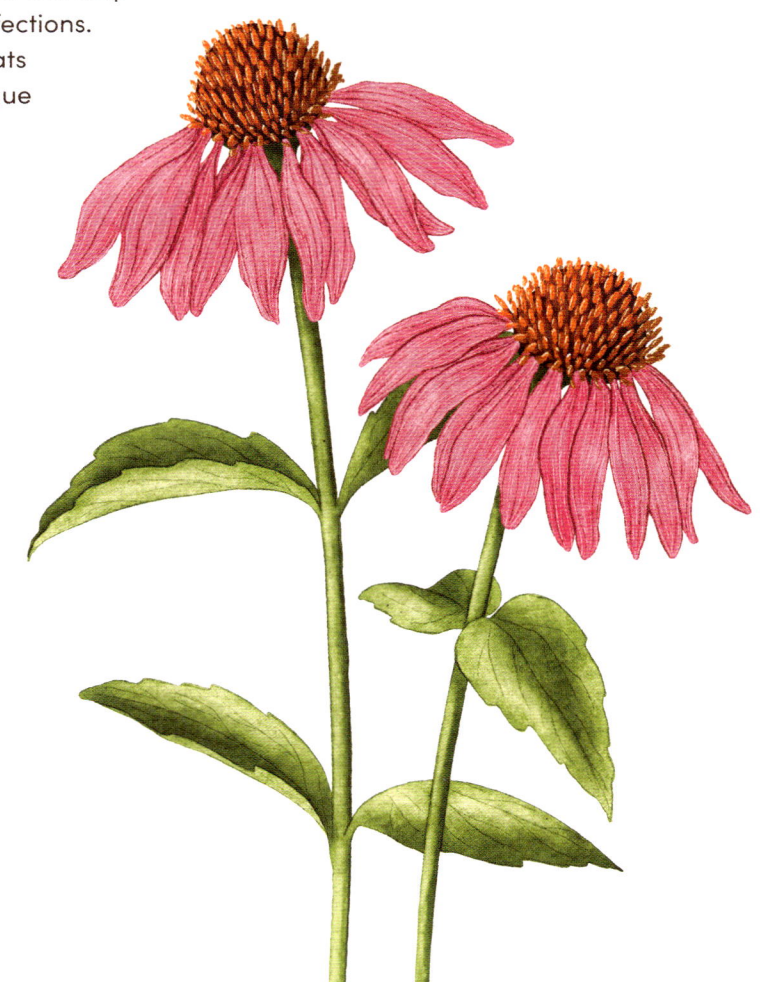

How to Grow:

 WHEN TO PLANT: Direct sow in fall for mild winter climates, or in late spring after the danger of frost has passed in colder climates. Start indoors 8–10 weeks before the last frost for transplanting in late spring.

 GROWS BEST FROM: Seed, transplant, or root division. Seed germination can be slow, but cold stratification improves this. Seeds can take 10–30 days to germinate, so many growers like to source live transplants or divide root systems from established echinacea plants to get a jump start. Transplants can establish quickly and are more likely to flower in the first or second year.

 SUN AND SOIL NEEDS: Full sun to partial shade. Tolerant of poorer soils, but thrives with moderate fertility. Regular moisture is needed when establishing young plants. Once mature, echinacea is drought tolerant.

 VARIETIES TO TRY: *Echinacea purpurea*, *Echinacea angustifolia*, and *Echinacea pallida*.

 SPACING: Space plants 18–24" apart to allow airflow and strong root growth. Echinacea patches will slowly expand each season, so plan for future spread.

 BLOOM TIME: From seed to bloom typically takes 2 years.

 HARVESTING TIPS: You can harvest small amounts of aerial parts (flowers and leaves) in the first year of growth, but it's best to wait until the second year. Year 3 is the threshold for beginning to harvest the roots. Waiting allows the plants to grow larger root systems that can handle some pruning for medicinal use.

GROWING TIP:

Echinacea can wane in productivity after 3–4 years. To continuously cultivate new plants, let some flower heads dry out fully and plant them in nearby soil. *Echinacea purpurea* is a flowering perennial that fits well into a cottage garden because of its upright, showy vertical stems and striking blooms.

How to Use:

 INFUSED OIL: Dried flowers and leaves can be infused for skin-healing salves.

 TINCTURE: 1 part fresh root to 2 parts 70% alcohol, or 1 part fresh aerial parts to 2 parts 50% alcohol, or 1 part dried root parts to 5 parts 60–70% alcohol. Fresh plant tinctures are considered most potent for acute immune support and lymphatic system cleansing.

 TEA: Steep 1–2 teaspoons dried aerial parts, covered, per 1 cup hot water for 10–15 minutes (fresh aerial parts contain a grassier, less palatable flavor, so dried is best). A stronger decoction is best when using the roots of the plants. For a root decoction, simmer 1 tablespoon dried root with 2 cups water for 20–30 minutes, covered. Strain and drink warm. This tea can help lessen the severity and duration of cold and flu symptoms, stimulate immune cells to help the body fight off pathogens, decrease inflammation, and soothe sore throats.

 POULTICE AND COMPRESS: Pulverized fresh roots or aerial parts can be applied as a poultice to bites, stings, or inflamed skin. A cold compress can be used as an antiseptic wound-healer and to reduce abscesses and boils.

General Safety:

TOPICAL USE: Generally safe, but may cause a mild rash on sensitive skin.

INTERNAL USE: Safe for short-term use but not recommended for long-term daily use. May interact with immunosuppressant drugs and other medications, making them weaker or stronger than intended. Those with autoimmune disorders should be careful with consumption of the roots, as they contain immune-stimulating properties. Using aerial parts can be a gentler way of supporting the immune system. Pregnant and nursing women should use caution and consult with their doctors.

HERBALIST TIP:

Echinacea is most effective when taken at the first signs of illness rather than as a long-term daily tonic. The root's herbal properties are stronger than the aerial parts, but it takes 2–3 years before root harvest, so many home herbalists use flowers and leaves in years 1 and 2 while waiting for roots to establish.

Elderberry

Sambucus nigra, Sambucus canadensis
Perennial in zones 4–9

This fast-growing shrub, producing clusters of creamy white flowers followed by purple-black berries, is long cherished for its immune-supporting properties and culinary uses.

Medicinal Properties:

TOPICAL: Elderberry's flowers soothe inflamed skin, sunburns, and minor wounds.

INTERNAL: Its flowers act as a diaphoretic, and they can treat fevers, colds, and congestion. The berries are rich in antioxidants and can help to shorten the duration of colds and flu.

ENERGETIC: Cooling, moistening.

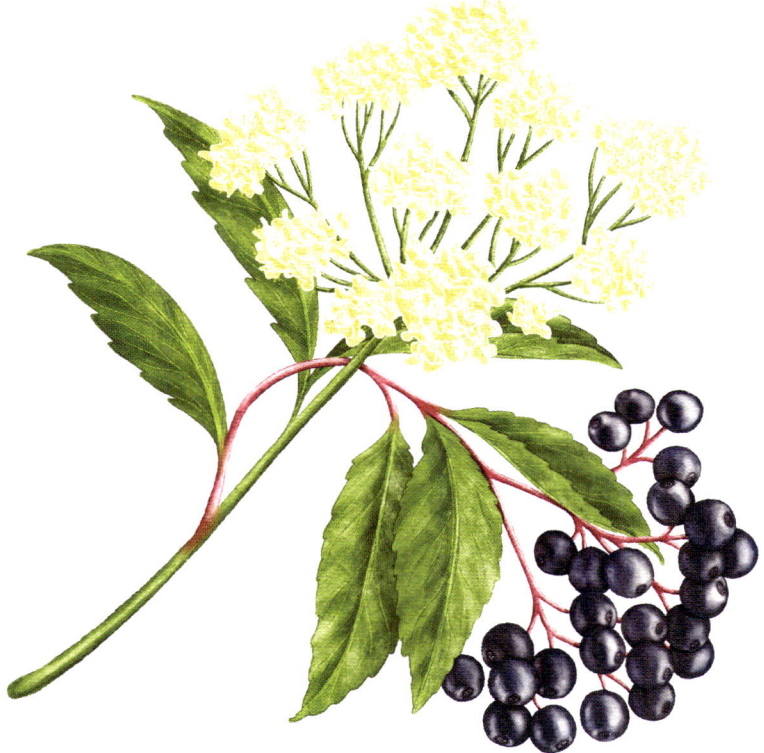

How to Grow:

 WHEN TO PLANT: Plant bare-root or potted shrubs in early spring after the last frost, or in fall in mild climates. (Bare-root herbs are cost-effective plants that have been dug up during dormancy [winter] and have had the soil rinsed from their roots.) These plants are usually younger than potted tree transplants but are very good for establishing multiple plants in the garden.

 GROWS BEST FROM: Rooted cuttings, bare roots, or nursery transplants. Elderberry can be grown from seed, but germination is slow and requires stratification. Hardwood or softwood cuttings root readily and are the easiest method. Bare-root plants can be sourced online easily, and local plant groups are a good source for cuttings.

 SUN AND SOIL NEEDS: Full sun, 6–8 hours or more, but can tolerate small amounts of shade. Moist, well-draining soil is optimal for growing, but elderberries are adaptable to poor conditions if given consistent moisture.

 VARIETIES TO TRY: York, Adams, Black Lace, and Haschberg.

 SPACING: Space shrubs 6'–10' apart, depending on the variety.

 BLOOM TIME: Elderberry shrubs transplanted from nursery stock (1–2 years old) can begin producing flowers and fruit within 1–2 years. Expect a reliable larger harvest by the second and third year after transplanting.

 HARVESTING TIPS: Harvest flowers in late spring to early summer, when clusters are fully open but not yet browning. Harvest berries in late summer to early fall when they are fully dark purple/black and plump.

GROWING TIP:

Elderberries are best grown with two plants near each other for cross pollination and better fruit set.

How to Use:

 INFUSED OIL: Not the typical use, but elderflowers can be infused into oil for soothing skincare products.

 TINCTURE: 1 part dried berries to 5 parts 40–50% alcohol. Used to shorten the length of a cold or viral illness.

 TEA: Steep 1–2 teaspoons fresh elderflowers per 1 cup water for 10–15 minutes for fevers, colds, and congestion. Fresh flowers have the best fragrance and flavor, but be sure to remove all stems before infusing, as they can be toxic. You can also simmer 2 teaspoons dried elderberries for 20 minutes to make a decoction that extracts the full medicinal properties of the herb for strong antiviral and immune support.

 POULTICE AND COMPRESS: Crushed fresh elderflowers can be applied as a poultice to inflamed or swollen areas. A cold compress soaked in elderflower tea can be used on the forehead and temples to reduce fever.

 SYRUP: Elderberries simmered and sweetened into syrup is a common immunity tonic.

⚠ General Safety:

TOPICAL USE: Generally safe for most skin types.

INTERNAL USE: Cook berries before use to neutralize toxins. Avoid raw berries and all leaves or stems. Elderflowers are considered safe in tea amounts for pregnant and nursing women, but elderberries should be used in moderation and always cooked. Elderberries can exacerbate autoimmune disorders and their symptoms, so those affected should use them with caution.

HERBALIST TIP:

Elderberry is best known for stimulating an immune response, so it can be especially useful at the early onset of viral infections. Harvest only the ripe, fully black berries. Unripe green berries can cause stomach upset. Freeze extra berries to have on hand year-round for making syrup or tea blends.

Elecampane

Inula helenium
Hardy perennial in zones 3–8

Elecampane is a tall, stately plant with large, rough leaves and bright yellow, sunflower-looking flowers. The roots are the main medicinal part.

Medicinal Properties:

TOPICAL: Used in infused-oil chest rubs for coughs and congestion.

INTERNAL: Expectorant, antimicrobial, bitter tonic, and carminative. Traditionally used for deep lung conditions as well as sluggish digestion.

ENERGETIC: Warming, drying.

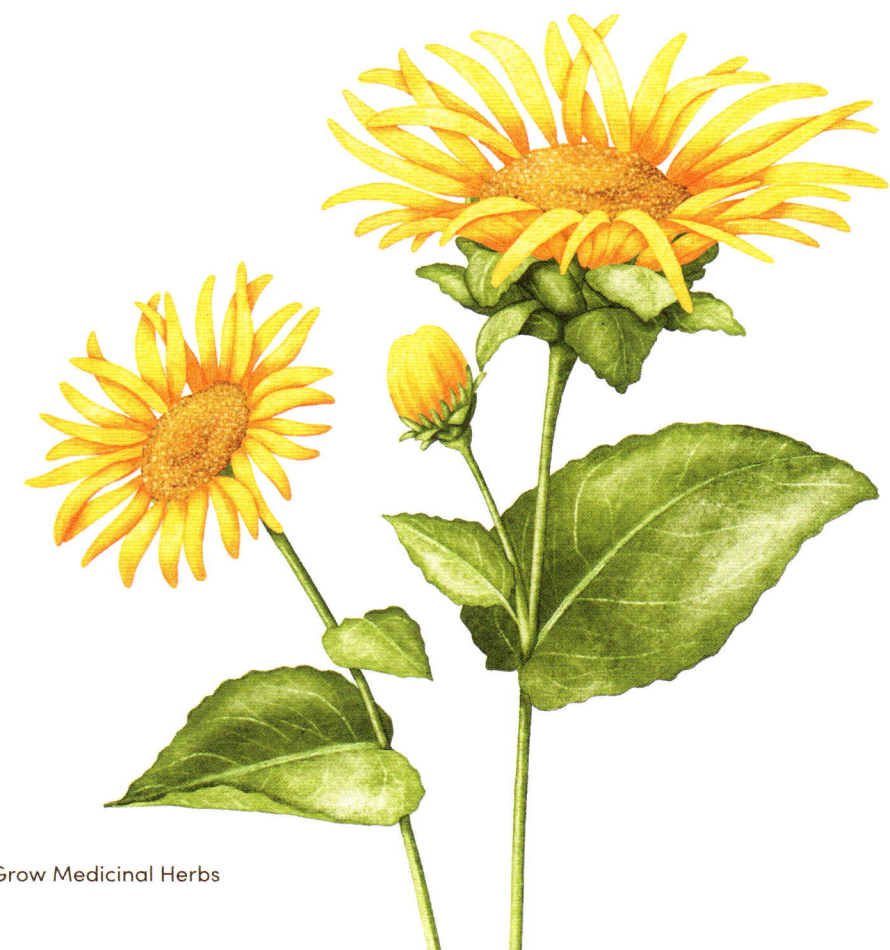

How to Grow:

 WHEN TO PLANT: Direct sow outdoors in fall in warmer winter regions as a wildflower, or in early spring in colder regions. You can also start indoors 6–8 weeks before the last frost.

 GROWS BEST FROM: Seed or root division. Seeds germinate slowly, sometimes taking 2–3 weeks to sprout. Transplants should be ready to plant outside 6–8 weeks after seeding. As a perennial, this herb can be divided by the root systems every 3–4 years to grow more plants.

 SUN AND SOIL NEEDS: Full sun to partial shade. Prefers deep, rich, moist, well-drained soils.

 VARIETIES TO TRY: Common elecampane, giant elecampane, and dwarf elecampane.

 SPACING: Space plants 24–30" apart. This herb has very large leaves (similar to a sunflower) that require space for airflow and proper growth. Plants can get 4–6' tall and grow in clumps that reach 2–3' wide once fully established.

 BLOOM TIME: Aerial parts (flowers, stems, and leaves) can be harvested in mid to late summer in the first year of growth, but roots should be harvested once the plant is 2 or more years old and established.

 HARVESTING TIPS: Peak root harvest is after the second year of growth.

GOOD TO KNOW:

The name elecampane comes from the medieval Latin name of the plant, *Enula campana*. Legend says Helen of Troy carried the plant with her, hence the species name *helenium*. It has a long reputation as a lung and digestive herb, and it has been used since Roman times in food and medicine.

How to Use:

 INFUSED OIL: Infused oil can be combined with beeswax for a lung congestion chest rub.

 TINCTURE: 1 part fresh root to 2 parts 55–70% alcohol, or 1 part dried root to 5 parts 50–60% alcohol. Used to break up wet, congested coughs and as a bitter tonic that stimulates sluggish digestion.

 TEA: Simmer 1–2 teaspoons dried root per 1 cup hot water for 10–15 minutes to address coughs and digestive sluggishness. Brewing longer, for 20–30 minutes, creates a standard decoction.

 POULTICE AND COMPRESS: Fresh elecampane poultices are not recommended. A weak tea soaked onto a towel for a compress can be used with caution to help with minor skin infections, fungal rashes, and eruptions.

 SYRUP: Combine a root decoction with honey for soothing coughs.

⚠ General Safety:

TOPICAL USE: Generally safe, but may irritate sensitive skin.

INTERNAL USE: Safe in moderate doses. Large amounts may cause nausea due to bitterness. Pregnant and nursing women should avoid strong medicinal doses, as this herb has the potential to stimulate the uterus. Avoid use if allergic to plants in the Asteraceae family.

HERBALIST TIP:

Elecampane is one of the best herbs for deep, chronic lung conditions—think phlegmy coughs that linger. Its warming, aromatic qualities both stimulate digestion and clear lungs, making it a classic dual-purpose bitter expectorant. Mixing an elecampane tincture with honey can help create a truly soothing herbal combination for the lungs while reducing the bitter strong flavors of this herb.

Fenugreek

Trigonella foenum-graecum
Annual

A clover-shaped legume with white or light yellow flowers, fenugreek is grown for its seeds and leaves and has been used in culinary and medicinal traditions for centuries. It has a distinctive maple syrup scent and is valued both as a kitchen spice and for its support of digestion.

Medicinal Properties:

TOPICAL: Used externally to soothe inflammation, boils, and sore muscles.

INTERNAL: Demulcent that soothes the gut and supports digestion, eases constipation, stimulates appetite, and helps regulate blood sugar and cholesterol. Traditionally used as a galactagogue to support lactation and ease menstrual discomfort.

ENERGETIC: Warming, moistening.

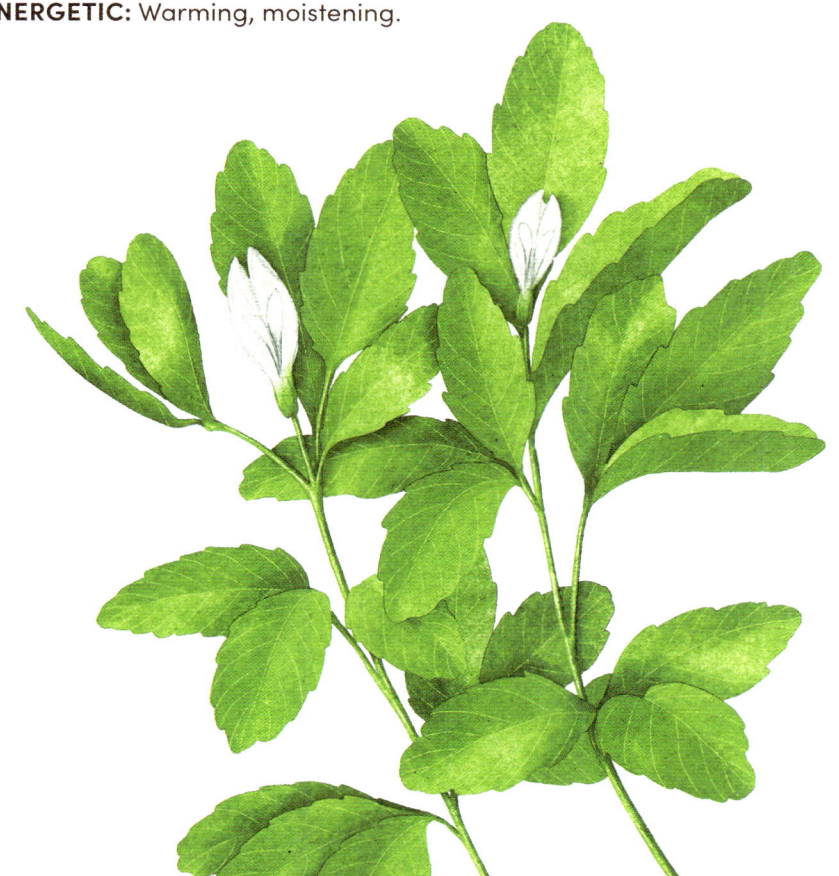

How to Grow:

 WHEN TO PLANT: Direct sow in early spring after the last frost, or in fall in mild climates. Prefers cooler weather.

 GROWS BEST FROM: Seed. Sow seeds ¼" deep into well-drained soil. Germination is quick, often within 3–5 days.

 SUN AND SOIL NEEDS: Full sun, 6–8 hours or more. Moderately fertile, well-drained soil is best for healthy growth. Fenugreek is a legume that can also help enrich the soil with nitrogen.

 VARIETIES TO TRY: Standard fenugreek and kasuri methi.

 SPACING: Sow seeds 2–3" apart in rows 6–8" apart. Plants grow 1–2' tall. Container friendly.

 BLOOM TIME: 90–110 days for seed harvest. Leaves can be harvested for use much earlier, 20–30 days after sowing.

 HARVESTING TIPS: Cut outer leaves as needed, leaving the central crown to regrow. Frequent harvesting encourages bushier growth. Pods will form after 60–75 days and should be ready to harvest in 90–110 days. Harvest when pods turn yellow-brown and begin to dry, but before they shatter and drop seeds.

GOOD TO KNOW:

Fenugreek's strong curry aroma can linger on the skin after heavy use. Using gloves while handling this herb can help avoid lingering smells.

How to Use:

 INFUSED OIL: Crushed seeds can be infused into oil and used topically for inflammation and muscle soreness.

 TINCTURE: Not typically tinctured for medicinal use.

 TEA: Steep 1 teaspoon dried seeds, lightly crushed, per 1 cup hot water for 10–15 minutes. Fenugreek has a slightly bitter maple flavor. Used in "mother's milk" tea blends to boost breast milk supply. Can also help relieve constipation and reduce blood sugar spikes when consumed alongside food.

 POULTICE AND COMPRESS: Ground, soaked seeds can be applied warm as a poultice to swellings, boils, or sore joints. Although not as effective, a hot compress made with fenugreek tea can provide similar benefits.

 ## General Safety:

TOPICAL USE: Generally safe, but may irritate sensitive skin.

INTERNAL USE: Generally safe in culinary and tea amounts. High doses may lower blood sugar and interact with diabetes medication or blood thinners. Not recommended during pregnancy in large amounts, as it may stimulate uterine contractions. Traditionally used to support lactation after birth, but may cause some gas and bloating in infants. Consult your healthcare provider before use.

HERBALIST TIP:

Soaking fenugreek seeds overnight makes them easier to digest and reduces bitterness in both culinary and medicinal uses. Toasting fenugreek seeds can also help reduce bitterness and bring out aromatic flavors in culinary use.

Feverfew

Tanacetum parthenium
Short-lived perennial in zones 4–9

This is a hardy herb with small, daisy-shaped white flowers and a strong, somewhat bitter scent. Feverfew has been long valued for its role in reducing headaches and migraines, as well as for calming inflammatory conditions.

Medicinal Properties:

TOPICAL: Soothes insect bites, minor wounds, and inflamed skin.

INTERNAL: May help prevent migraines, reduce inflammation, ease arthritis, and calm fever (hence its name).

ENERGETIC: Cooling, drying.

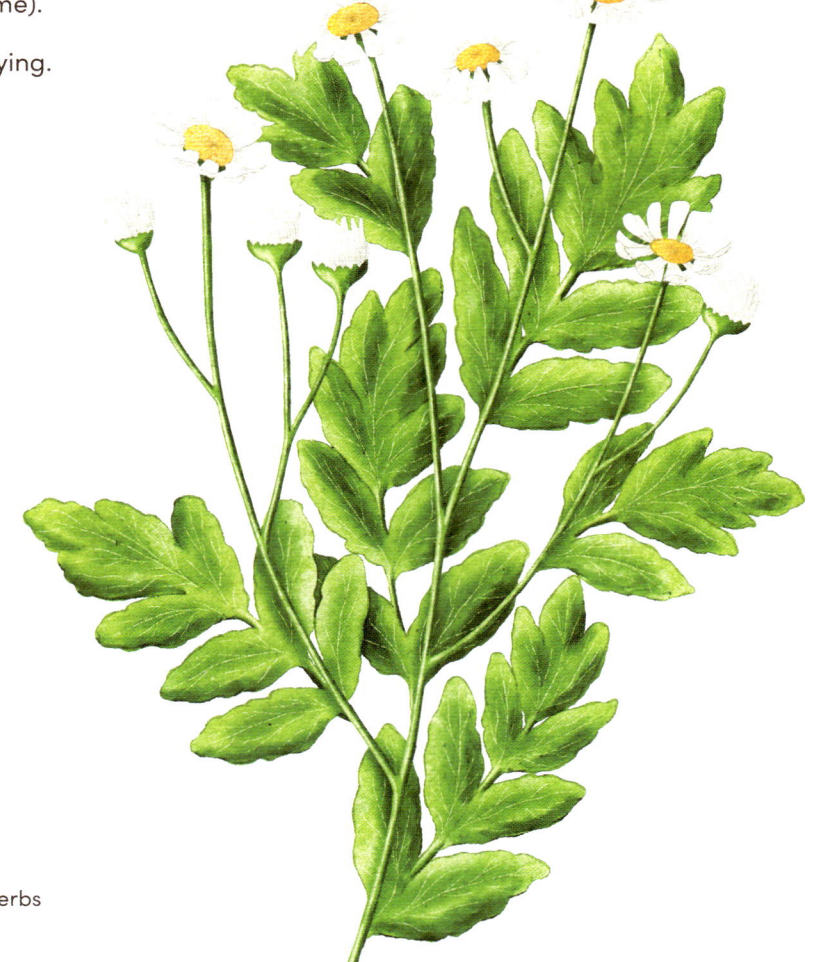

How to Grow:

 WHEN TO PLANT: Direct sow in spring after the danger of frost has passed, or start indoors 6–8 weeks before last frost.

 GROWS BEST FROM: Seed or transplant. Seeds need light to germinate, so press into the soil surface rather than covering. Germination takes 10–14 days.

 SUN AND SOIL NEEDS: Full sun, 6–8 hours or more, and well-drained soil. Tolerant of poorer soils but thrives with moderate fertility. Regular moisture is needed when establishing young plants. Once mature, semi-regular, deep waterings are preferred.

 VARIETIES TO TRY: Standard feverfew, Golden Feverfew, and double-flowered varieties

 SPACING: Space plants 12–18" apart to allow airflow and prevent mildew. Feverfew plants can get quite large when in full bloom, so give ample space for young plants to grow in. Fully grown plants can get up to 3' wide and 24" tall once flowers are in full bloom.

 BLOOM TIME: 70–90 days from seed to initial blooms. Flowers throughout summer with regular deadheading.

 HARVESTING TIPS: Harvest young leaves throughout the growing season for tinctures and fresh preparations. Pick flowers at peak bloom for drying or fresh use.

GOOD TO KNOW:

Feverfew has been called the "medieval aspirin" for its ability to reduce headache pain and inflammation. It's most effective when used regularly as a preventative herb, rather than at the onset of a migraine. Although a perennial, it may behave as a self-seeding annual in colder climates (zones 3–4) or climates with extreme heat (zones 9b–10).

How to Use:

 INFUSED OIL: Dried leaves and flowers can be infused for topical anti-inflammatory use.

 TINCTURE: 1 part dried herb to 5 parts 40% alcohol is often used for migraine prevention.

 TEA: Steep 1 teaspoon dried flowers, covered, per 1 cup hot water for 10–15 minutes (fresh parts have a stronger flavor that is often less palatable, so it's best to use dried). Feverfew has a very strong and bitter flavor, so it is often blended with other herbs. Used as a prophylactic for migraines, for digestive support, and for fever reduction.

 POULTICE AND COMPRESS: Crushed fresh leaves can be applied as a poultice directly to insect bites or inflamed areas. A cold compress can be made with feverfew tea to reduce localized joint swelling and pain.

⚠ General Safety:

TOPICAL USE: Can irritate sensitive skin.

INTERNAL USE: Not recommended for pregnant women, as it may stimulate the uterus. Breastfeeding mothers should avoid it due to limited safety data. Prolonged fresh leaf chewing can cause mouth ulcers.

HERBALIST TIP:

Feverfew works best as a preventive for migraines when taken regularly in small amounts, rather than waiting for pain to start.

Garlic

Allium sativum

Perennial in zones 3–8 (usually grown as an annual crop)

Garlic is a hardy bulb crop in the allium family, treasured for both culinary and medicinal uses. Though technically a perennial, it's usually grown as an annual and harvested for its bulbs.

Medicinal Properties:

TOPICAL: Used for earaches and fungal skin infections.

INTERNAL: Antimicrobial that can help with urinary tract issues, antiviral, antifungal, and antiparasitic. Supports cardiovascular health, reduces fluid retention, helps lower blood pressure, and boosts immune defense.

ENERGETIC: Warming, drying.

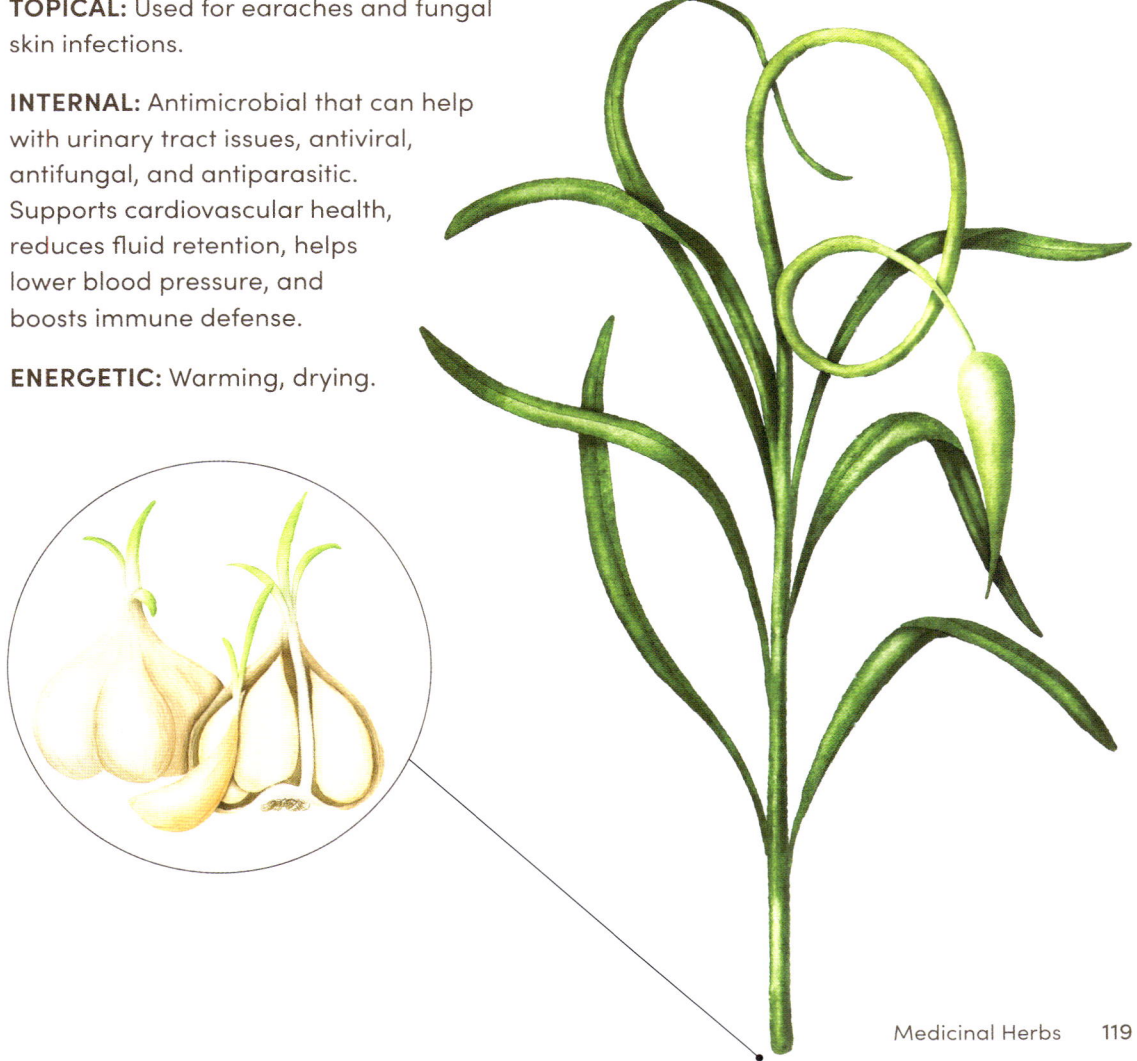

How to Grow:

 WHEN TO PLANT: Plant garlic cloves in the fall (October–November in most regions) for harvest the following summer. In order to form full heads that contain multiple cloves, garlic must go through a period of cold weather. This process is called "vernalization." In warmer climates, you may need to chill cloves in your fridge for 6 weeks before planting to mimic a winter "season" and encourage full heads of garlic to form by the following summer.

 GROWS BEST FROM: Individual cloves (not seed). Separate cloves from the bulb and plant with the pointed end up. Each clove of garlic will turn into a full head of garlic that contains multiple cloves of its own by the end of the process.

 SUN AND SOIL NEEDS: Full sun, 6–8 hours or more. Prefers well-drained, very fertile soil enriched with compost amendments. Avoid soggy soil to prevent rot. Mulch garlic cloves at least 3–4" deep with dead leaves or straw mulch in the winter to avoid early sprouting in hotter climates and fully frozen cloves in colder climates.

 VARIETIES TO TRY: Hardneck garlic (e.g., Rocambole, Purple Stripe), softneck garlic (e.g., silverskin, artichoke), and elephant garlic.

 SPACING: Plant cloves about 6" apart. Keep rows about 12" apart for airflow and ease of weeding. Set cloves 2–3" deep, pointed end facing up. Garlic takes up very little space in a garden, so consider adding it along borders or in open spaces.

 BLOOM TIME: Typically 8–9 months from cloves to harvest.

 HARVESTING TIPS: Harvest when ½–⅓ of the leaves have turned brown. Cure bulbs in a dry, shaded, well-ventilated place for 2–3 weeks before storing. Store cured bulbs in a cool, dry location for several months (softnecks last longest).

GOOD TO KNOW:

Garlic is one of the oldest known medicinal plants, with records of use dating back more than 5,000 years. Hardneck garlic produces scapes (curly flower stems) in spring, which are edible and delicious when sautéed or pickled. Softneck garlic does not form scapes, but stores longer.

How to Use:

 INFUSED OIL: Garlic can be infused into oil for earaches or fungal skin infections.

 TINCTURE: 1 part fresh chopped garlic to 2 parts 95% alcohol makes a highly potent antimicrobial extract. It can be very effective in safer, small doses diluted in water or added to honey before taking.

 TEA: Steep 2–3 slices garlic (or what you can tolerate) per 1 cup hot water for 5–10 minutes, then sweeten with honey and add lemon juice to taste. Garlic tea steeped with honey and lemon is traditional for colds and flu.

 POULTICE AND COMPRESS: Crushed fresh garlic can be applied as a poultice to help infection, but dilute with a skin-safe oil to avoid skin irritation. A compress is not typically used with garlic.

 General Safety:

TOPICAL USE: Can irritate or burn skin if applied directly. Always dilute.

INTERNAL USE: Generally considered safe in culinary amounts. High doses may cause digestive upset and interact with blood thinners. Generally safe in food amounts for pregnant and nursing women, but medicinal doses should be used with caution.

HERBALIST TIP:

Vinegar infused with garlic and other aromatic, powerful herbs is a traditional herbal preparation known as an oxymel. Fire cider (see Chapter 3) is one of these recipes. It allows the freedom to add any immune-boosting or -modulating herbs to the vinegar before sweetening it with honey to help make the preparation more palatable. In general, garlic works best as a medicine when it's crushed and allowed to sit for 10–15 minutes before use. This waiting period activates allicin, the compound responsible for much of garlic's antimicrobial and immune-supporting properties.

Ginger

Zingiber officinale
Perennial in zones 9–12

Ginger is a tropical "clumping" perennial with slender, reed-like stems and narrow lance-shaped leaves that grow from knobby underground rhizomes.

Medicinal Properties:

TOPICAL: Helps with arthritic pain, muscle soreness, and stiffness.

INTERNAL: Increases circulation. Carminative that helps with gas and nausea. Diaphoretic that promotes perspiration to help reduce cold symptoms, warms the body to reduce chills, and relieves congestion.

ENERGETIC: Warming, drying.

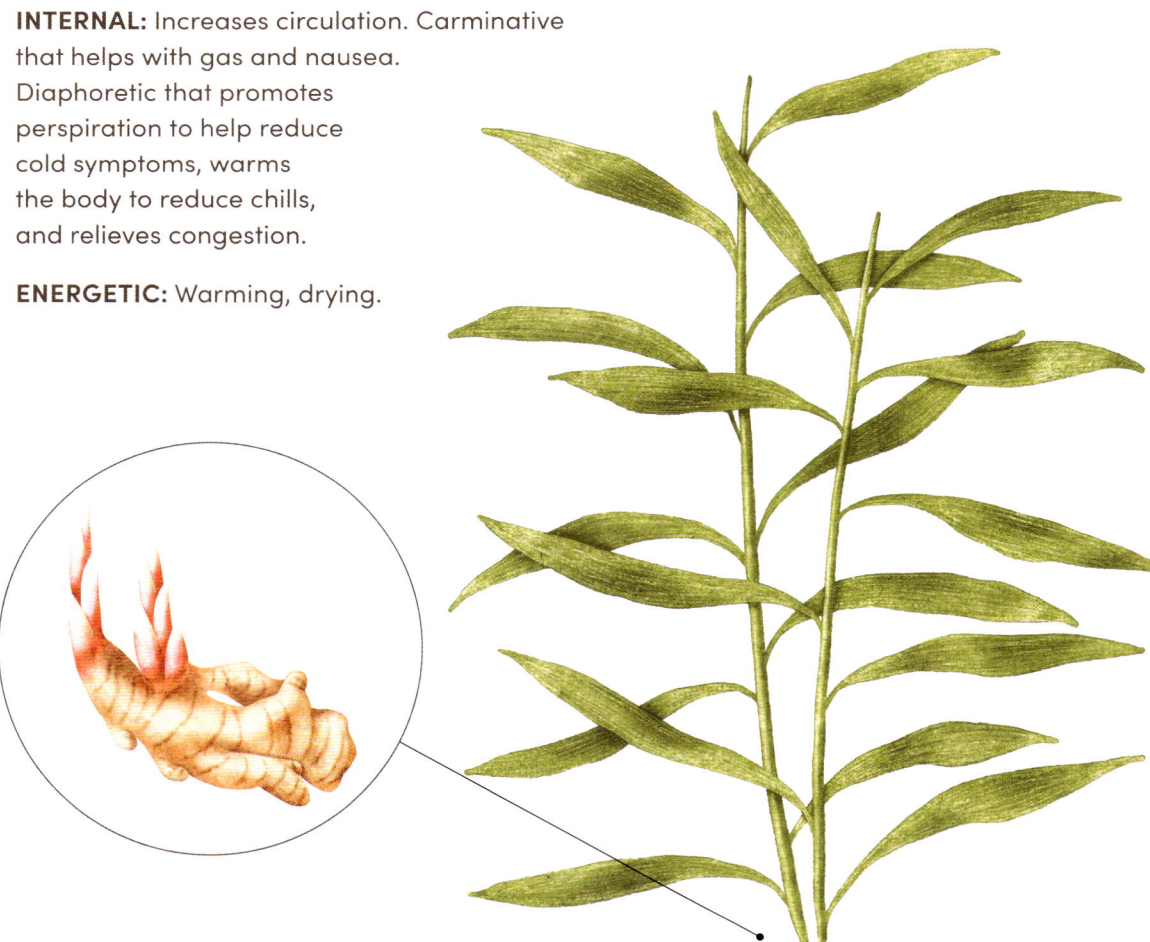

How to Grow:

 WHEN TO PLANT: Plant ginger rhizomes directly outdoors once soil temps are consistently above 60°F. (This is always in early summer, after the threat of last frost has passed and nights have warmed a bit.) In tropical areas, ginger can be planted year-round. In colder climates, you can start sprouting the rhizomes inside under grow lights to transplant outside after frost has passed.

 GROWS BEST FROM: Rhizome. You can sprout or directly sow rhizomes and they will eventually grow larger. Choose rhizomes with at least one bud, since that is where the sprouts form. These can be dug up and divided each year to make more plants. Ginger rhizomes have natural segments or joints. To divide these rhizomes, look for a piece with at least one healthy bud, or "eye," and a few roots attached. You can gently break them apart at a natural joint. Each segment can be replanted separately and will grow into a new plant.

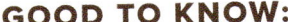

GOOD TO KNOW:

Ginger is a "companion herb" that is often added to herbal blends to increase absorption and effectiveness of other herbs. For example, ginger stimulates bile that can help the body absorb curcumin, the active constituent in turmeric.

 SUN AND SOIL NEEDS: Partial shade to filtered sun. In very hot climates, ginger does best with afternoon shade or dappled light to prevent scorching. It needs loose, rich, loamy soil that drains well. Ginger does not like compacted heavy clay soils, and rhizomes will rot if waterlogged. On the other hand, soil that's too dry slows rhizome development. Ginger grows shallowly, so raised beds and wide containers work well.

 VARIETIES TO TRY: Chinese ginger, yellow ginger, Jamaican ginger, Queensland ginger, and shampoo ginger.

 SPACING: Sow rhizomes 8–12" apart or 12–18" apart if planting in rows. Plant rhizomes 2–4" deep with the buds' "eyes" facing upward. Containers should be at least 12" wide per plant. Wide, shallow containers are best for rhizomes to spread horizontally.

 BLOOM TIME: Baby ginger (the young, pale rhizomes) are usually ready 4–5 months after planting. Fully mature ginger take 8–10 months of warm weather after planting to be ready.

 HARVESTING TIPS: Harvest rhizomes when leaves start yellowing and dying back in late fall. You can save some rhizomes to dry and store for replanting in the spring.

How to Use:

 INFUSED OIL: Ginger root (rhizome) can be gently warmed in a carrier oil to create an infused warming massage oil.

 TINCTURE: 1 part fresh herb to 2 parts 70% alcohol, or 1 part dried herb to 5 parts 60–70% alcohol. Used for reducing nausea and symptoms of motion sickness; lessening gas, flatulence, and bloating; stimulating digestion; and easing headaches, migraines, and muscle or joint pain.

 TEA: Steep 1 teaspoon dried root per 1 cup boiling water, covered, for 10 minutes. Or, simmer two or three ¼"-thick slices of fresh ginger per 1 cup water in a pot for 10–15 minutes to make a stronger decoction. Fresh ginger is more helpful for nausea, but dried or frozen ginger can be spicier and more stimulating/warming.

 POULTICE AND COMPRESS: Grated ginger can be applied as a poultice to encourage circulation and reduce localized pain. A warm compress can be made from ginger tea and applied to sore muscles and joints.

 BATH SOAK: Fresh ginger or ginger powder added to bathwater or a foot bath can create a stimulating and warming soak for treating colds, chills, and sore muscles.

⚠ General Safety:

TOPICAL USE: Well tolerated by most people, but those with sensitive skin may have irritation, redness, or burning with use. Avoid use on broken skin or open wounds.

INTERNAL USE: Generally safe in culinary and tea amounts for most adults and children. Can cause heartburn, stomach upset, or diarrhea in high doses. Avoid consuming ginger if taking a blood-thinning medication, as ginger may increase bleeding risk. Keep in mind that it can also lower blood pressure and blood sugar. Considered safe in moderate tea/food amounts for pregnant or nursing mothers.

HERBALIST TIP:

When making ginger tea for respiratory support, be sure to cover the tea while it is steeping. The steam holds volatile oils that help open the sinuses and ease breathing. You can even sip while inhaling the steam to combine both internal and inhaled use benefits! Also, freezing fresh ginger can help break down plant cell walls, allowing more flavor to be extracted during the tea-brewing process.

Holy Basil

Ocimum tenuiflorum

Annual in most zones, short-lived perennial in zones 10–12

Holy basil, a warm season, shrubby plant with purple flowers, is also known as tulsi.

Medicinal Properties:

TOPICAL: Mild antimicrobial that is used in skin washes and poultices for minor fungal or bacterial irritation.

INTERNAL: Adaptogen (aids the body's stress response) and supports adrenal health. Calms the nervous system while gently increasing mental clarity. Gentle expectorant that opens airways and dries mucus. Digestive stimulant. Promotes gentle sweating. Antioxidant rich.

ENERGETIC: Mildly warming, drying.

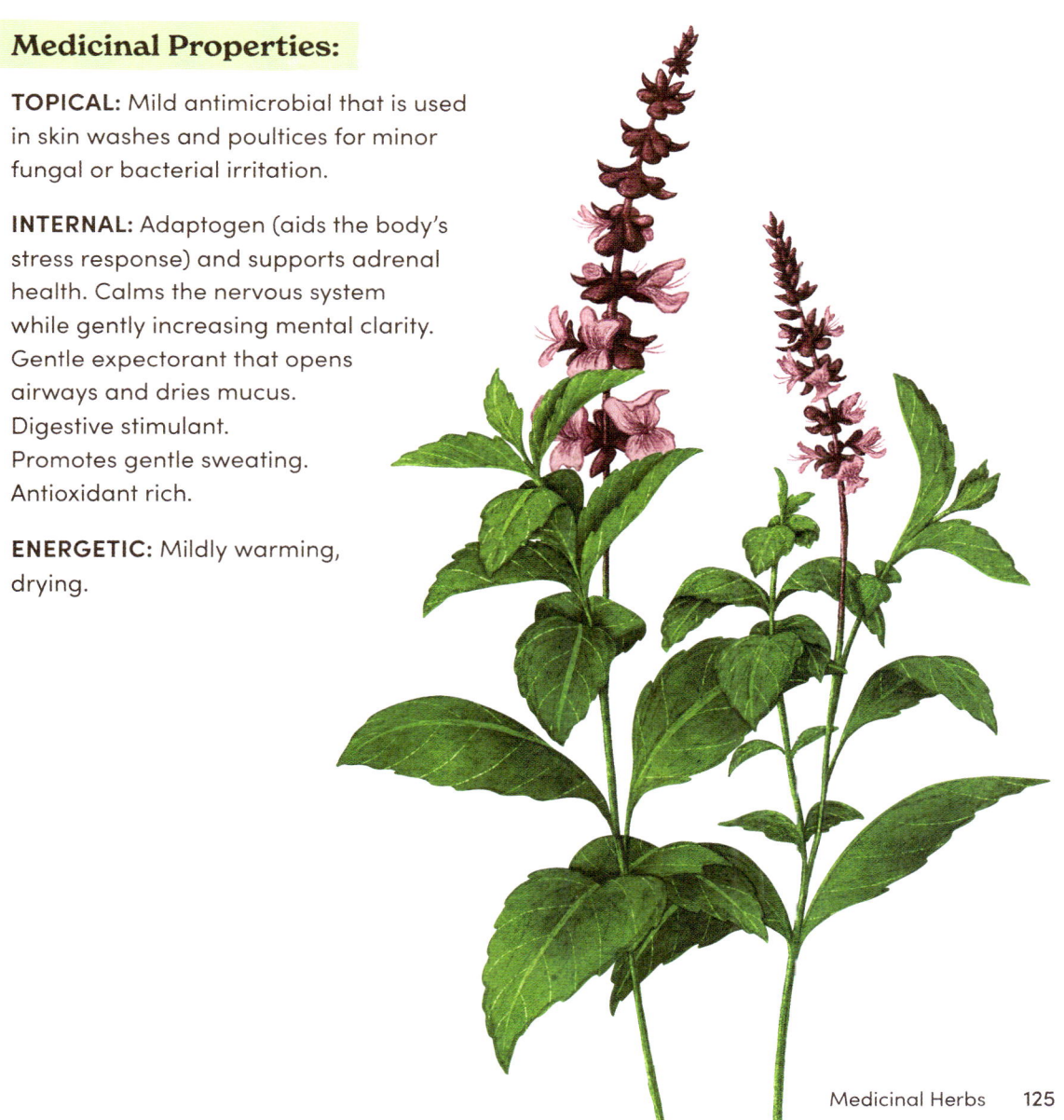

How to Grow:

 WHEN TO PLANT: Sow or transplant after the danger of frost has passed and soil has warmed to at least 60°F. In mild climates, start seeds indoors 4–6 weeks before last frost.

 GROWS BEST FROM: Seed or transplant. Sow seeds on the soil surface or no more than ¼" deep. Germinates in 5–14 days with warmth.

 SUN AND SOIL NEEDS: Full sun, 6–8 hours or more. Prefers fertile, well-draining soil with moderate moisture.

 VARIETIES TO TRY: Krishna tulsi, Rama tulsi, Kapoor tulsi, and Vana tulsi.

 SPACING: Space plants 12–18" apart. Plants do well grown in containers or garden beds. Prune the stems often to create bushier growth.

 BLOOM TIME: 60–75 days from seed to harvest. Produces flowers in the summer. Pinch back blooms to encourage more leaf growth.

 HARVESTING TIPS: Begin harvesting leaves once plants are at least 6–8" tall. Remove the top 4–6" of the plant to use. Leaves bruise easily and lose aroma quickly after harvest, so they're best used fresh or dried promptly. For teas, pick just before it flowers for strongest potency.

GOOD TO KNOW:

Holy basil, or tulsi, is deeply woven into Indian culture, and it is often grown in courtyards and temples for its spiritual significance. The plant releases its aroma when touched, attracting pollinators, like bees, but deterring some pests.

How to Use:

 INFUSED OIL: Not typically made with this herb.

 TINCTURE: 1 part fresh aerial parts (flowers, stems, and leaves) to 2 parts 50–60% alcohol. Used as an adaptogenic herb to reduce stress, anxiety, and mental fatigue.

 TEA: Steep 1–2 teaspoons dried leaves, or ¼ cup fresh leaves, per 1 cup hot water for 10–15 minutes for stress relief, immune support, and respiratory health.

 POULTICE AND COMPRESS: Crushed fresh leaves can be applied as a poultice or compress to help with antibacterial and antifungal treatments.

 General Safety:

TOPICAL USE: Well tolerated by most people.

INTERNAL USE: High concentrations not recommended for pregnant or nursing mothers. Some light culinary-based consumption is tolerated, but always consult a doctor.

HERBALIST TIP:

Holy basil is often dried and used in tooth powders and mouth rinses in tea form. Tooth powder is an alternative to toothpaste, made by grinding dried holy basil leaves into a fine powder. It is usually blended with other herbs, like neem or licorice, or with charcoal and clays. To use, dip a damp toothbrush into the powder or rub directly onto gums and teeth with a clean finger. You can also use holy basil to make a skin toner.

Horehound

Marrubium vulgare

Hardy perennial in zones 4–9

This gray-green, wooly-leaved plant in the mint family has square stems and clusters of small white flowers.

Medicinal Properties:

TOPICAL: Not commonly used externally.

INTERNAL: Bitter tonic, expectorant, and carminative. Traditionally used for coughs, colds, bronchitis, indigestion, nausea, and a loss of appetite.

ENERGETIC: Warming, drying.

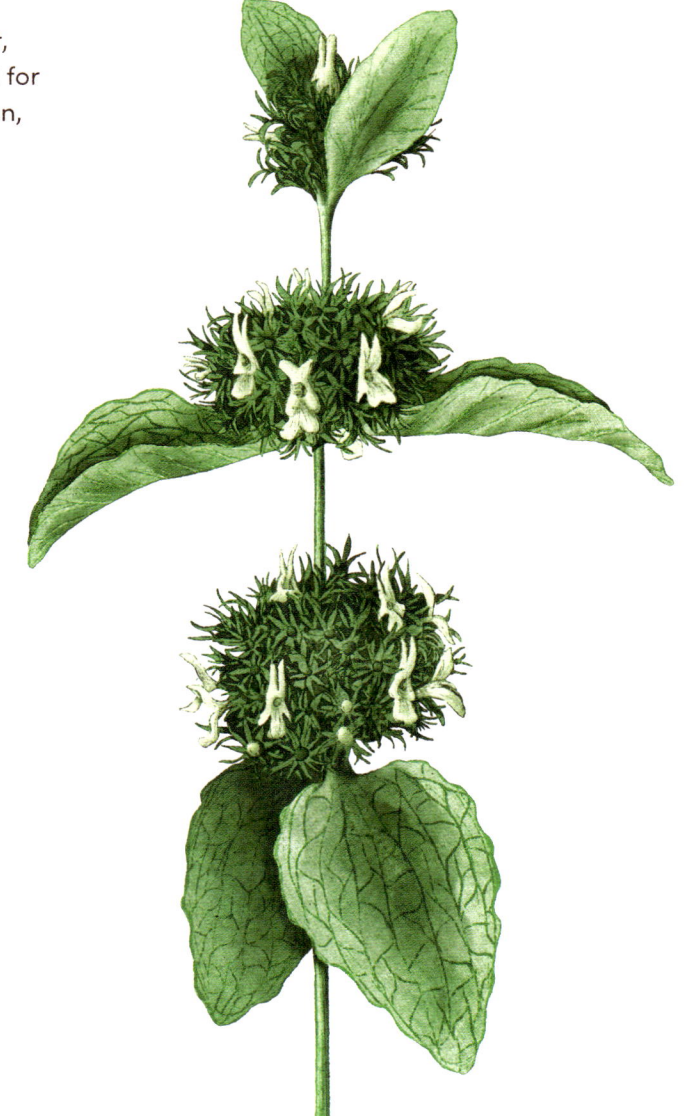

How to Grow:

 WHEN TO PLANT: Sow outdoors in spring after the last frost, or indoors 6–8 weeks before last frost.

 GROWS BEST FROM: Seed or stem cuttings. Self-seeds easily. Seeds are very small, like mint seeds, and should be sowed on the surface of the soil. Germination can take 7–14 days, but sometimes longer. Seedlings take 4–6 weeks to reach transplant size. Cuttings can be taken throughout the growing season and rooted in water for transplanting into soil to create more plants.

 SUN AND SOIL NEEDS: Full sun, 6–8 hours or more, but some after-noon shade in southern regions is tolerated. Prefers dry, sandy soil or poor soils. Very drought tolerant once established.

 VARIETIES TO TRY: Common white horehound, creeping horehound, and black horehound.

 SPACING: Space plants 12–18" apart. This herb grows in rounded clumps that can eventually spread, but it can be a slow process unless the plant is allowed to reseed in place. Container friendly.

 BLOOM TIME: Typically 60–70 days after seeding.

 HARVESTING TIPS: Peak harvest of aerial parts (flowers, stems, and leaves), for strongest bitterness and medicinal power, arrives once plants are 10" tall and in full bloom. As a perennial, it returns yearly and self-seeds readily. Cut back the plant after bloom to encourage fresh growth.

GOOD TO KNOW:

Horehound is the classic herb behind horehound candy and cough drops. The bitterness is key to its expectorant and digestive actions—the strong taste itself stimulates the body's reflexes for saliva, bile, and mucus production.

How to Use:

 INFUSED OIL: Not typically made with this herb.

 TINCTURE: 1 part fresh herb to 2 parts 50–60% alcohol, or 1 part dried herb to 5 parts 40% alcohol. Either mixture can be used for coughs and digestion.

 TEA: Steep 1–2 teaspoons dried herb per 1 cup hot water for 15 minutes. Tea is very bitter, so it is often blended with honey or licorice. To extract the medicinal benefits of the fresh leaves, it's best to make a decoction of 1 cup fresh horehound leaves to 4 cups water, simmered for 15–30 minutes, covered. Used as an expectorant that can break up and thin mucous, soothe the airways, and calm rattling coughs.

 POULTICE AND COMPRESS: A poultice of fresh crushed horehound leaves can be applied to slow-healing sores, ulcers, and minor wounds. A compress made with a horehound decoction can give similar benefits but is less commonly used.

General Safety:

TOPICAL USE: Generally safe, but always do a patch test to avoid skin irritations.

INTERNAL USE: Safe in moderate doses. Bitterness may cause nausea in excess. Pregnant and nursing women should avoid strong medicinal doses, as this herb is a traditional emmenagogue. May lower blood pressure slightly. Use cautiously with heart medications.

HERBALIST TIP:

Horehound shines as a classic lung herb. It can help treat stubborn, phlegmy coughs where mucus is hard to expel. You can make throat lozenges/cough drops with a horehound infusion or decoction cooked with sugar or honey at a high temperature until the mixture thickens. Dry and shape into drops.

Horsemint

Monarda punctata

Short-lived perennial in zones 4–9

This herb is a square-stemmed mint family plant with whorls of white to pale purple dotted bracts that sometimes have a cream or yellow hue.

Medicinal Properties:

TOPICAL: Antimicrobial and antiseptic. Treats fungal infections and skin eruptions.

INTERNAL: Carminative and antimicrobial. Also an expectorant and diaphoretic. Relieves colds, coughs, sore throats, indigestion, and intestinal cramping.

ENERGETIC: Warming, drying.

GROWING TIP:

The showy flower bracts make horse-mint not only medicinal but also a pollinator magnet in the garden. As a short-lived perennial, it may persist 2–3 years, but most can renew themselves by self-seeding to start over again.

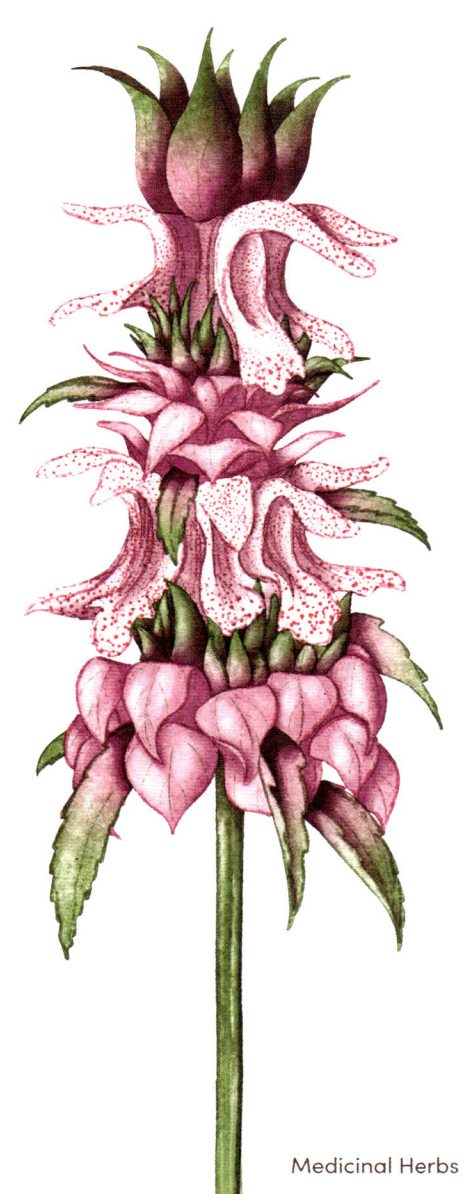

How to Grow:

 WHEN TO PLANT: Sow seeds outdoors in fall as a wildflower in more mild winter climates, or sow them outdoors after the last frost in early spring in colder winter climates. Or, sow at both times to have better chances at germination and patch establishment.

 GROWS BEST FROM: Seed or root division. Seeds are very small and should be surface sown, as they need light to germinate. Scatter seeds in 4" pots and keep the top of the soil moist. Germination can take from 10–21 days. Clumps of established plants can be dug up to replant roots else-where for more plants.

 SUN AND SOIL NEEDS: Full sun, 6–8 hours or more, helps with strong blooms. Prefers well-drained, sandy, or rocky soil.

 VARIETIES TO TRY: Common spotted horsemint and wild lemon mint.

 SPACING: Sow seeds in clumps 12–18" apart to allow for future spreading. Plants grow 2–3' tall.

 BLOOM TIME: The plant takes 90–120 days to bloom.

 HARVESTING TIPS: You can begin a light leaf harvest at 80–90 days after seeding, once plants reach 10–12" tall. Gather aerial parts (leaves and flowering tops) just as plants begin to bloom for peak oil content.

HERBALIST TIP:

Think of horsemint as a wild "prairie thyme." It is stronger than many mints and has excellent antiseptic power. It's best used for short-term, acute conditions, like colds or digestive infections, rather than in long-term daily tonics.

How to Use:

 INFUSED OIL: Not typically made with this herb.

 TINCTURE: 1 part fresh herb to 2 parts 50–60% alcohol, or 1 part dried herb to 5 parts 40–50% alcohol. Tincturing fresh preserves more of the mint family's volatile properties. Used in small doses for digestive upset, colds, and infections.

 TEA: Steep 1 teaspoon dried leaves and flowers, or 2 teaspoons fresh leaves, per 1 cup hot water, covered, for 10 minutes. Horsemint has a strong thyme flavor, and is often blended with other herbs. This herb is very strong, so a small amount goes a long way even when using fresh leaves. Used to relieve gas and bloating, break a fever, and dry up mucous.

 POULTICE AND COMPRESS: Crushed fresh aerial parts can be applied as a poultice directly to wounds, fungal rashes, or skin eruptions. Tea brewed from the aerial parts can be used as an antifungal and antiseptic compress/rinse.

 STEAM INHALATION: Add 1–2 tablespoons dried horehound leaves (or ¼ cup fresh, lightly crushed) to a bowl of hot water. Tent your head with a towel and inhale the vapors for 5–10 minutes to help open sinuses, loosen mucus, and clear congestion.

⚠ General Safety:

TOPICAL USE: Generally safe. Essential oil form may cause skin irritation if too concentrated.

INTERNAL USE: Use in moderation. Can cause nausea or stomach upset in high doses and should be avoided by pregnant and nursing women.

Lavender

Lavandula angustifolia
Perennial in zones 5–9 (variety dependent)

This hardy, sun-loving, semi-woody perennial with silvery green foliage and fragrant purple flower spikes is cherished for its calming aroma, medicinal qualities, and beauty.

Medicinal Properties:

TOPICAL: Mild antimicrobial. Soothing, mild antiseptic. Reduces itchiness and redness from insect bites and rashes. Soothes sore muscles and joint stiffness.

INTERNAL: Nervine that promotes restful sleep. Carminative that eases gas, bloating, and nervous stomach. Can help ease tension headaches and migraines.

ENERGETIC: Cooling, drying.

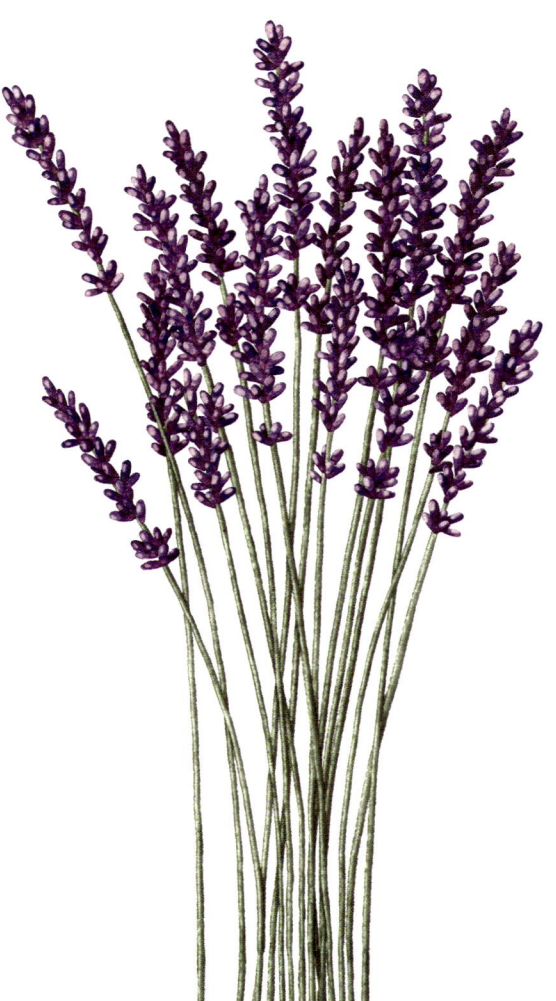

GOOD TO KNOW:

Lavender's name comes from the Latin word *lavare*, meaning "to wash," because it was used in Roman baths and laundry for cleansing and fragrance. Today, it's one of the most studied herbs for stress relief and remains a cornerstone of both herbal medicine and aromatherapy.

How to Grow:

 WHEN TO PLANT: Sow or transplant after the danger of frost has passed. In mild climates, start seeds indoors 6–8 weeks before last frost.

 GROWS BEST FROM: Stem cuttings or transplants, though it takes 10–12 weeks for young plants to be strong enough for transplant. It can be grown from seed as well, but germination can be slow (up to 30 days) and erratic. Lavender seeds do best with cold stratification to improve sprouting rates. Cuttings can be made from the semi-woody portions of the plants in late spring or early summer.

 SUN AND SOIL NEEDS: Full sun, 6–8 hours or more, helps it bloom better and lowers risk for fungal disease. Lavender needs very well-draining soil that is sandy or gravelly. Avoid heavy clay or soggy soil. Drought tolerant once established. Prefers infrequent, deep watering.

 VARIETIES TO TRY: English lavender, French lavender, Spanish lavender, and lavandin.

 SPACING: Space plants 18–24" apart to allow proper airflow. Plants can get from 12–24" tall and 18–24" wide depending on the cultivar.

 BLOOM TIME: Lavender grown from seed typically won't give much usable bloom the first year. From transplants, expect usable flowers in 3–6 months with strong yields starting in year 2.

 HARVESTING TIPS: Harvest when about half of the flower buds are open for best balance of fragrance, color, and oil content. Never cut into the woody base, as it weakens the plant.

How to Use:

 INFUSED OIL: Oil infusions can be used in salves and balms to help soothe burns, rashes, and insect bites.

 TINCTURE: 1 part fresh herb to 2 parts 50–60% alcohol, or 1 part dried herb to 5 parts 40% alcohol, can provide concentrated relief for anxiety, tension headaches, and digestive complaints.

 TEA: Steep 1 teaspoon dried flowers, or 1 tablespoon fresh flowers, per 1 cup hot water, covered, for 5–10 minutes. Lavender tea has a strong floral flavor on its own, so it's often blended with supporting herbs, such as lemon balm, mint, or chamomile, in order to improve taste and to enhance its relaxing, digestive, and calming effects.

 POULTICE AND COMPRESS: Used as a compress for headaches, cramps, or localized pain.

 STEAM INHALATION: Add a handful of fresh flowers/stems, or 2–3 tablespoons dried, to a bowl of hot water. Tent your head with a towel and inhale vapors for 5–10 minutes. Keep eyes closed to avoid irritation. Used to promote calmness, restful sleep, and respiratory relief.

⚠ General Safety:

INTERNAL USE: Generally safe in culinary, tea, and topical use. May irritate skin. Essential oil extractions can burn skin if not properly diluted in carrier oils. Culinary use is generally seen as safe for pregnant or nursing women, but high medicinal doses should be avoided.

HERBALIST TIP:

Lavender's essential oils are volatile. Always cover your cup while steeping to keep the beneficial oils from evaporating. Uncover only when you're ready to sip, so you capture both the flavor and the relaxing aromatics.

Lemon Balm

Melissa officinalis
Perennial in zones 4–9

This fragrant, perennial mint-family herb is known for its bright green, lemon-scented leaves.

Medicinal Properties:

TOPICAL: Antiviral compounds. Helpful with reducing cold sores. Soothes bug bites or minor rashes.

INTERNAL: Calming effect on the central nervous system. Nervine for mild anxiety, tension, and headaches. Helps promote restful sleep. Carminative that eases nausea, gas, and bloating. Aids in memory and focus.

ENERGETIC: Cooling, slightly drying.

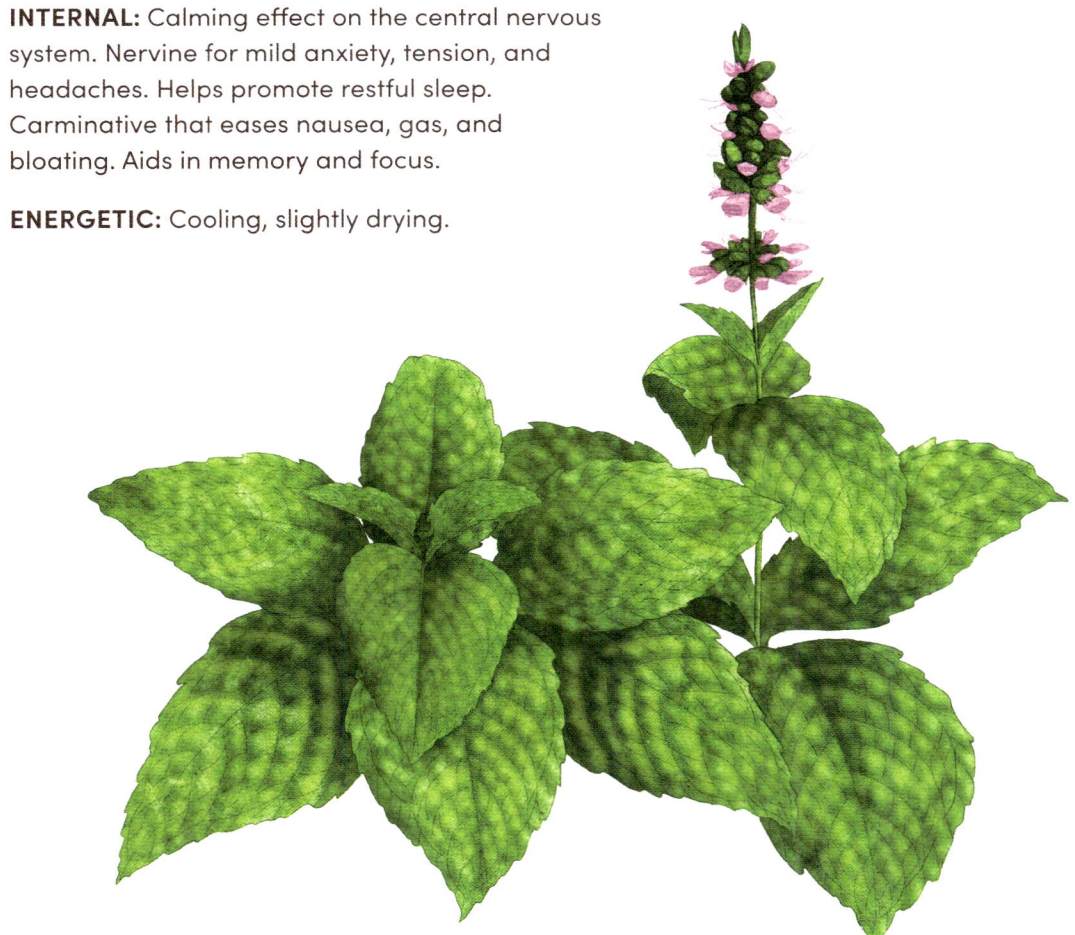

How to Grow:

 WHEN TO PLANT: Sow or transplant after the danger of frost has passed. In mild climates, start seeds indoors 6–8 weeks before last frost.

 GROWS BEST FROM: Seed or transplant. Sow seeds on the soil surface and gently press in. Keep soil moist and warm for better germination (the seeds are tiny, so the process can be difficult). Seeds need light to germinate. Germination can take from 7–14 days.

 SUN AND SOIL NEEDS: Full sun to partial shade. Lemon balm needs more shade in hotter climates, specifically in the afternoon. Prefers fertile, well-draining soil with moderate and consistent moisture.

 VARIETIES TO TRY: Common Good, Quedlinburger Niederliegende, Citronelle, Compacta, and All Gold Bright.

 SPACING: Most gardens don't need multiple lemon balms, but be sure to space this plant out from other plants to allow airflow, as fungal issues can be a risk. It will grow to be 18–24" tall, and it can spread aggressively through runners underground. Container growing will avoid spreading.

 BLOOM TIME: 70–90 days from seed to harvest. Produces flowers in the summer.

 HARVESTING TIPS: Begin harvesting leaves once plants are at least 8–12" tall. The best flavor and potency is just before plants start to flower.

GOOD TO KNOW:

Lemon balm has a long-held reputation for being a "gladdening herb." French monks in the seventeenth century used it in tonics and perfumes to lift the spirit. The flowers of the plant are irresistible to bees, helping lemon balm to earn its name, Melissa, which comes from *mélissa*, the Greek word for "honeybee."

How to Use:

 INFUSED OIL: Dried leaves can be infused into oils, salves, and balms for topical use.

 TINCTURE: 1 part fresh herb to 2 parts 95% alcohol; tincture fresh to preserve the volatile citrusy oils. Used for easing nervous tension, anxiety, and irritability. Can also uplift mood, ease insomnia, and calm a nervous stomach by easing stomach cramps, nervous indigestion, gas, and bloating. Also used for its antiviral properties.

 TEA: Steep ¼ cup fresh leaves, or 2 teaspoons dried leaves, per 1 cup hot water, covered, for 10–15 minutes. Lemon balm is a slightly sweet and lemony herb that blends well with the flavors and medicinal properties of chamomile. Used for reducing stress and anxiety, and easing gas, bloating, indigestion, and nausea.

 POULTICE AND COMPRESS: Used in poultices to help with viral skin issues or cold sores. Used with compresses to help with tension headaches or sunburn recovery.

⚠ General Safety:

TOPICAL USE: Well tolerated by most people, but volatile oils can irritate sensitive skin.

INTERNAL USE: High concentrations are not recommended for pregnant or nursing women. Some light culinary consumption is tolerated, but always consult a doctor first. Avoid combining with other sedative medications. Those with an underactive thyroid might need to avoid regular usage of lemon balm, as it can calm or slow down an overactive thyroid.

HERBALIST TIP:

For cold sores, use a cold lemon balm compress multiple times a day to reduce duration of outbreak.

Lemongrass

Cymbopogon citratus

Perennial in zones 9–11 (variety dependent)

A tall, clump-forming grass with a fresh, lemony scent, lemongrass is prized for its culinary, medicinal, and aromatic uses. It is valued in the garden for both its flavor and its natural pest-repelling qualities.

Medicinal Properties:

TOPICAL: Antimicrobial that is deodorizing and insect repelling; provides muscle and joint relief.

INTERNAL: Mild diuretic and digestive aid that can help reduce nausea; offers calming stress relief, immune support, and fever relief.

ENERGETIC: Cooling, drying.

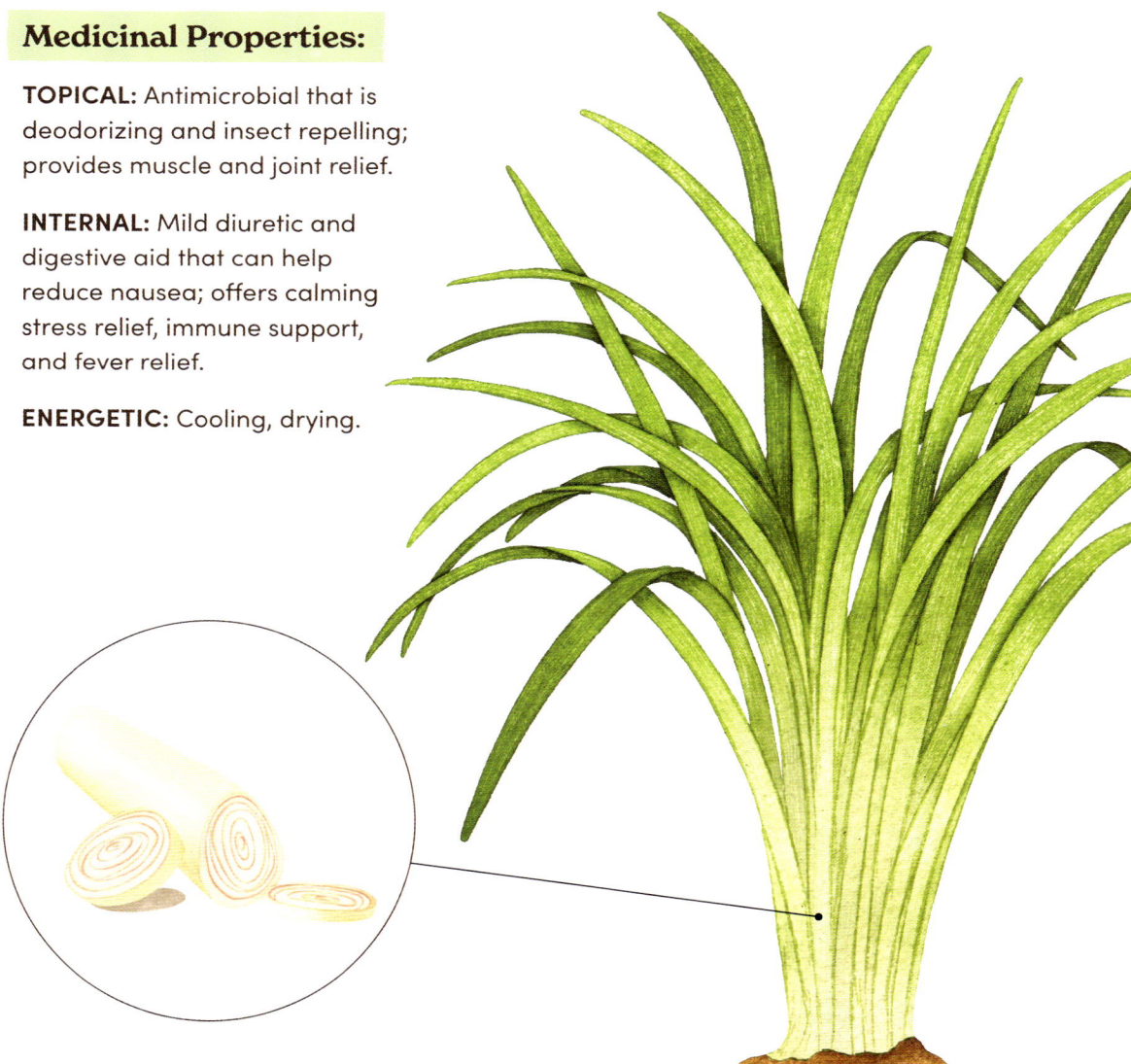

How to Grow:

 WHEN TO PLANT: Sow or transplant after the danger of frost has passed. In mild climates, start seeds indoors 6–8 weeks before last frost (expect 14–21 days to sprout).

 GROWS BEST FROM: Root division or stalk cuttings. It can be grown from seed as well, but germination is a bit slower, and soil must be 70–75°F. Place fresh stalks that have been pulled from the base of the plant (where the plant meets the soil) into a cup of water on a windowsill or under a grow light. Once roots form, transplant into soil.

 SUN AND SOIL NEEDS: Lemongrass thrives in tropical climates and with full sun, 6–8 hours or more. It will grow in shadier spots, but will take longer to establish thick stalks for culinary uses. Lemongrass can tolerate lower-quality soil, but it does better with slightly acidic amended soil (regular compost additions can help). Once established, the plants can tolerate some drought conditions, but lack of water can increase toughness of the stalks and reduce flavor.

 VARIETIES TO TRY: West Indian lemongrass, East Indian lemongrass, and citronella grass.

 SPACING: Space plants 24–36" apart to allow clumps to expand. Lemongrass can grow large, both in height and circumference. The leaves of lemongrass can irritate skin, so avoid planting this herb near walkways/pathways.

 BLOOM TIME: Light harvest 90–120 days from seed (3–4 months). For full-sized stalks with usable bulbs, expect 4–6 months from seed. It will also take 4–6 months to harvest established divisions or root cuttings.

 HARVESTING TIPS: Begin cutting outer stalks once plants are 12–18" tall, leaving central stalks to keep growing. Peak flavor comes from the bulb end of mature stalks, but the leaves also contain medicinal value.

GROWING TIP:

In the garden, lemongrass doubles as an ornamental grass and natural insect deterrent thanks to its high citral content. A single healthy clump can produce dozens of stalks in a season. Its lush, fountain-like foliage makes a striking border plant. If you're in zone 8 or colder, plant lemongrass in a large container so you can bring it inside before a frost. Lemongrass actually handles being trimmed back and over-wintered indoors quite well.

How to Use:

 INFUSED OIL: Oil infusion is not the typical use for extracting medicinal properties from lemongrass, although some antimicrobial properties can be useful topically as hydrosols and essential oil extractions.

 TINCTURE: 1 part fresh herb to 2 parts 95% alcohol; tincture fresh to preserve the volatile oils. Provides concentrated relief for digestive upset and anxiety, and offers immune support.

 TEA: Steep 1–2 teaspoons dried leaves, or 1 fresh stalk cut into pieces, per 1 cup hot water, covered, for 10 minutes. Fresh or frozen lemongrass contains more of the flavor and medicinal properties, so it is preferred for use in tea. Used for aiding in digestion and inducing sweating to help break fevers during illness.

 POULTICE AND COMPRESS: Used in poultices to help with insect bites, fungal skin issues, and localized muscle aches. Used in compresses to aid in fever reduction, headaches, generalized muscle soreness, and calming.

 STEAM INHALATION: Add a handful of fresh leaves, or 2–3 tablespoons dried leaves, to a bowl of hot water. Tent your head with a towel and inhale vapors for 5–10 minutes. Keep eyes closed to avoid irritation. Used for headache relief, mental stimulation, and respiratory cleansing.

⚠ General Safety:

TOPICAL USE: Use any essential oil infusions carefully, because they can irritate sensitive skin.

INTERNAL USE: Generally safe in culinary and tea amounts for most adults and children. Large medicinal doses could cause stomach upset and increased urination. Culinary use is generally seen as safe for pregnant or nursing women, but high medicinal doses should be avoided due to possible uterine-stimulating effects.

HERBALIST TIP:

Use fresh lemongrass for the brightest flavor and strongest aroma. Dried leaves lose potency quickly. To preserve flavor for tea blends, freeze fresh stalks and leaves for later use.

Licorice Root

Glycyrrhiza glabra
Long-lived perennial in zones 7–10

Licorice root is a tall, luminous plant with pinnate leaves (on either side of the stem, in opposite pairs), pale purple to blue flowers, and long, fibrous, sweet-tasting roots.

Medicinal Properties:

TOPICAL: Used for soothing inflamed skin or ulcers.

INTERNAL: Demulcent, expectorant, adrenal tonic, and anti-inflammatory. Used to treat dry coughs, gastritis, ulcers, and adrenal fatigue, and to balance strong herbal formulas.

ENERGETIC: Cooling, moistening.

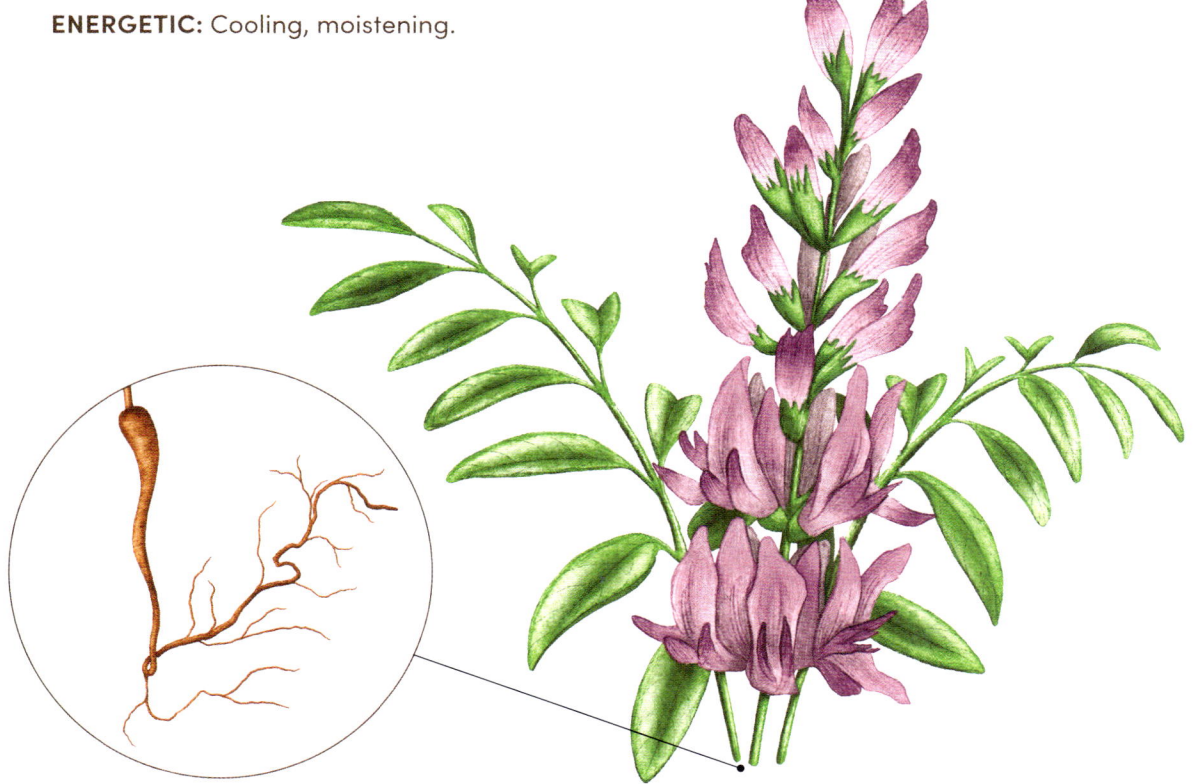

How to Grow:

 WHEN TO PLANT: Start seeds indoors in spring, then transplant after frost.

 GROWS BEST FROM: Rhizome cuttings, which are easier and more reliable than seeds for getting new plants started. To divide the root clumps, dig up portions of the plant's root system in early spring or fall when the plant is still dormant. Plant in large raised beds to create an easier root-harvesting system. Take portions of the clumps that have new sprouts or growth on them and replant elsewhere to get more plants. Seeds are difficult to germinate and benefit from roughing their outer coating to increase germination rates. Germination can take 14–28 days.

 SUN AND SOIL NEEDS: Full sun, 6–8 hours or more. Deep, somewhat sandy soils that have some balanced fertility are best, as licorice needs space for its long roots.

 VARIETIES TO TRY: Common licorice and Chinese licorice.

 SPACING: Space rhizome cuttings 18–24" apart. Licorice spreads slowly underground at first, but over the course of 5–6 years, it can form large colonies, especially in sandy loam where rhizomes travel easily. It is not invasive like mint, but it does gradually colonize an area underground.

 BLOOM TIME: Licorice can take 2–3 full growing seasons to mature enough to flower. In ideal conditions, you may see blossoms in year 3, but often it's closer to year 4 or 5 before reliable flowering occurs.

 HARVESTING TIPS: Leaves can be lightly harvested in the first year and can provide a more gentle version of the root's properties. In the fall of the third or fourth year, you can dig up a section of the root system of the plant to use medicinally.

GOOD TO KNOW:

Licorice root is up to 50 times sweeter than sugar due to a component called glycyrrhizin, yet it does not spike blood sugar. In Chinese medicine, it's considered a harmonizing herb that blends formulas and balances stronger herbs. Deglycyrrhizinated licorice is a root extract that has had most of the compound glycyrrhizin removed in order to reduce the risk of blood pressure and potassium side effects. Tinctured forms of licorice root contain the most concentrated amount of glycyrrhizin, so acute use with contraindications is suggested.

How to Use:

 INFUSED OIL: Licorice root can be infused for soothing irritated skin.

 TINCTURE: 1 part dried root to 5 parts 50–60% alcohol. Used for balancing adrenal stress and loosening mucus.

 TEA: Simmer 1 teaspoon dried root for 15–20 minutes as a decoction. Use as a naturally sweet way to soothe coughs and digestion.

 POULTICE AND COMPRESS: Best used as a compress with the cloth soaked in licorice root decoction and applied warm for chest discomfort and inflammation. A poultice is not typically made with licorice root.

 SYRUP: Combine a root decoction with honey for soothing dry coughs and sore throats.

 General Safety:

TOPICAL USE: Generally safe.

INTERNAL USE: Safe in moderate doses, but excess or long-term use can cause water retention, high blood pressure, and lowered potassium. Avoid use alongside diuretics, corticosteroids, or heart/blood pressure medications. Pregnant and nursing women should avoid strong medicinal doses because safety is not fully established.

HERBALIST TIP:

Dried root powder can be added to capsules or blended with other herbs to help balance out their energetics and flavor. Licorice can taste somewhat sweet and should be used in small doses, making it a great harmonizing herb.

Marshmallow Root

Althaea officinalis
Hardy perennial in zones 3–9

This tall, upright plant has soft, velvety leaves and pale pink to white hibiscus-like flowers. Its roots, leaves, and flowers are medicinal.

Medicinal Properties:

TOPICAL: Soothes inflamed or dry skin. Used to treat burns, rashes, and wounds.

INTERNAL: Demulcent, emollient, expectorant. Supports respiratory health. Soothes both digestive tract and urinary tract irritation. Can help ease a sore throat. Can also be used for soothing digestive discomfort in pregnancy and supporting breast milk production.

ENERGETIC: Cooling, moistening.

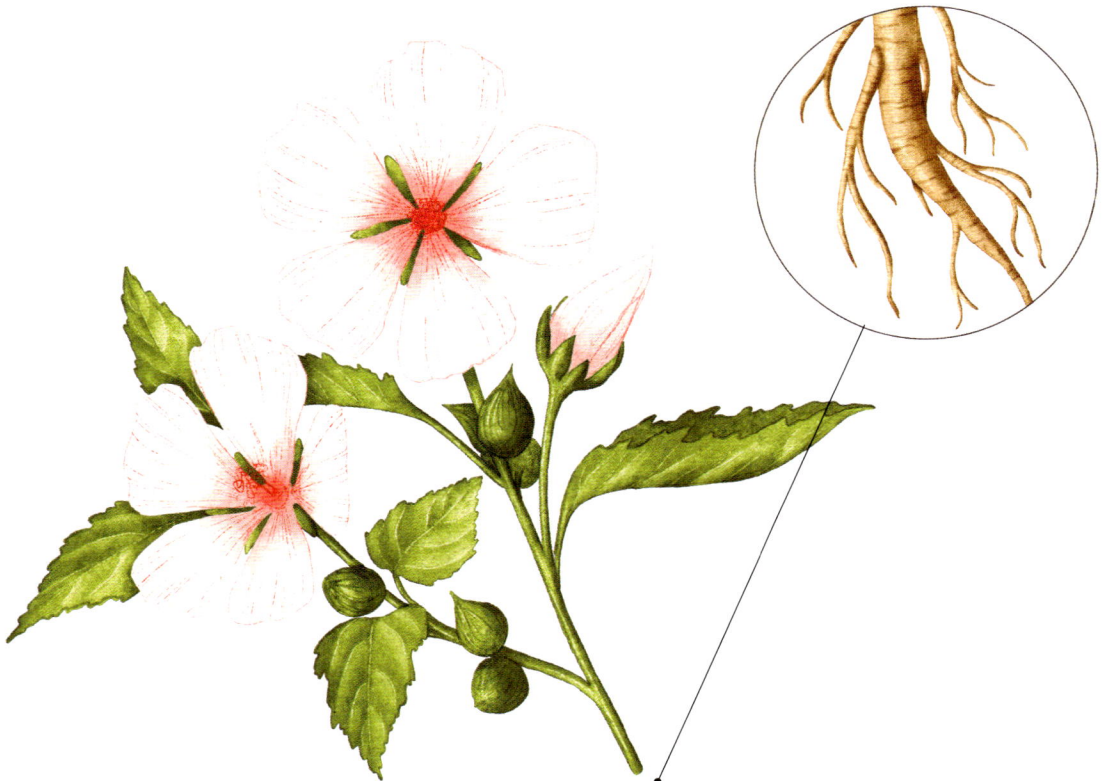

How to Grow:

 WHEN TO PLANT: Direct sow in the fall in milder winter climates to get plants established before the first frost. Direct sow after the last frost in colder winter climates.

 GROWS BEST FROM: Seed, but can also be propagated from root division in the spring every 3–4 years. Seeds benefit from 2–4 weeks of stratification to increase germination rates. Germination can take 14–21 days. Seedlings take 6–8 weeks to establish before being ready to transplant.

 SUN AND SOIL NEEDS: Full sun to partial sun. Prefers moist, rich, well-draining soil. Regular watering is essential for these plants.

 VARIETIES TO TRY: Common marshmallow, globe mallow, rose mallow, and rockrose.

 SPACING: Space plants 18–24" apart as plants grow upright and do not sprawl. The average marshmallow plant can get 3–5' tall, so planting this herb on the back edge of garden beds is best.

 BLOOM TIME: Marshmallow usually blooms in its second year, after overwintering (growing through the winter as a dormant perennial) and establishing roots. Blooms will usually show from June to August, producing soft pink, hibiscus-like flowers.

 HARVESTING TIPS: Leaves and flowers can be harvested lightly in the first year once plants are well established, at 90–120 days. Roots are best harvested in the fall of the second or third year, after plants have developed stronger roots.

GOOD TO KNOW:

The marshmallow plant is the original source of the marshmallow confection. Today's candy no longer contains the herb, but the plant remains a staple in herbal teas, syrups, and lozenges for coughs and digestive complaints. Ancient recipes blended root mucilage (a gel-like substance) with honey for soothing sore throats.

How to Use:

 INFUSED OIL: Use the root or leaves to infuse oil for soothing skin preparations.

 TINCTURE: Not typically used as a tincture.

 TEA: Steep 1–2 tablespoons dried root in a jar, covered with cold water, for several hours for mucilage-rich tea. For warm tea infusions, opt for room temperature or slightly warm water to extract as many benefits from the root as possible without degrading muci-lage. Used for soothing dry coughs, gastritis, stomach ulcers, acid reflux, heartburn, and the urinary tract. This tea can also ease constipation.

 POULTICE AND COMPRESS: Crushed fresh leaves or moistened powdered root can be applied as a poultice to burns, wounds, or insect bites. The powdered-root poultice can also be used to draw out splinters and boils. A compress made from cooled marsh-mallow root or leaf tea can be used to soothe sunburns, eczema, psoriasis, and dermatitis.

 SYRUP: A root decoction combined with honey can soothe coughs and sore throats.

⚠ General Safety:

TOPICAL USE: Very safe and gentle.

INTERNAL USE: Generally safe, even for children and elders. Safe in food and tea amounts for pregnant and nursing women.

HERBALIST TIP:

Marshmallow root contains mucilage, which is slippery and soothing to irritated tissues. Heat can break down this mucilage, reducing its soothing qualities. For the strongest extract of these properties, steep marshmallow root in cold water for several hours.

Milky Oats

Avena sativa
Annual

This is the common oat plant, but harvested at the "milky stage," when immature oat seeds exude a white, milky latex when squeezed.

Medicinal Properties:

TOPICAL: Oatstraw or ground oats are used in baths for itchy, inflamed skin.

INTERNAL: Nervine, demulcent, nutritive, and restorative. Supports issues with stress, burnout, and nervous exhaustion.

ENERGETIC: Cooling, moistening.

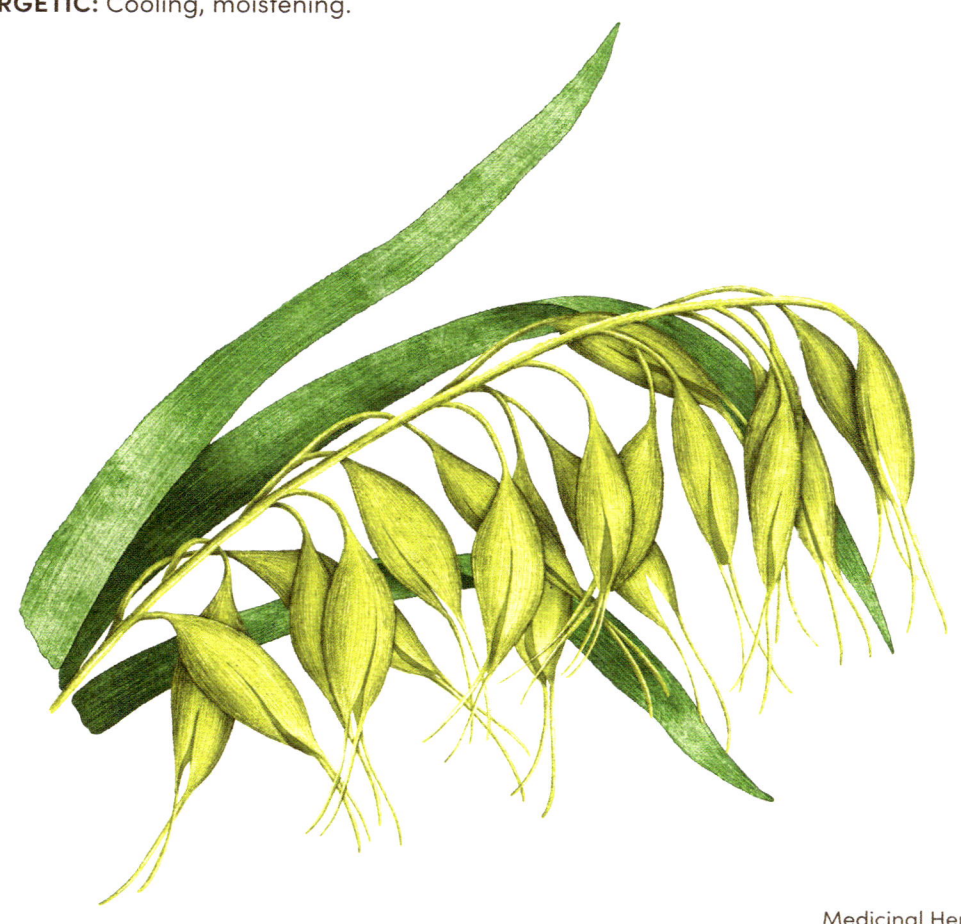

How to Grow:

 WHEN TO PLANT: Direct sow by broadcasting in rows, or as a cover crop in fall in milder winter climates and in early spring in colder winter climates.

 GROWS BEST FROM: Seed; does not transplant well. Broadcast seed and rake in, or sow ½–1" deep. Seeds take 7–10 days to germinate. The first stage of growth is the leafy grass stage that lasts 4–6 weeks.

 SUN AND SOIL NEEDS: Full sun, 6–8 hours or more. Prefers cool temps, fertile loamy soil, and consistent moisture.

 VARIETIES TO TRY: Common oat and hull-less oat.

 SPACING: Sow seeds in rows 6–8" apart. Grows as a tall grain in fields or patches.

 BLOOM TIME: The plants take 60–75 days to reach the milky stage after sowing. It can take 90–110 days for seed heads to mature, and stalks can be harvested for mineral-rich oatstraw. Full maturity of plants is usually at the 120-day mark if grown for food oats.

 HARVESTING TIPS: To harvest the milky oats at the correct time, keep an eye on the bulging of the oat "pods" on the fully formed oat stalks around the 60-day mark. Stalks and leaves must still be green, not brown or yellowing. To test the milky oats, pinch or press a pod between your thumbnail and fingertip. If a white, latex-type liquid oozes out, this is the "milk" stage. This stage only lasts 5–7 days. Since the milky oats will lose some of their properties if they dry out, freezing or tincturing the fresh harvest immediately is a best practice. You can harvest the entire plant at this same stage, while it's still mostly green. Cut the green stems into small pieces and dry them at very low temps (95°F or lower) to preserve the medicinal properties.

GOOD TO KNOW:

Milky oats are not the same as the mature oat grain. The milky stage lasts about a week, so harvesting at the right time is key. Fresh tincturing is ideal, since drying reduces the potency of the latex-rich seed juice. Oatstraw utilizes all the aerial parts of the plant and can be harvested after the milky oat seed heads are gathered, giving the oat plant two medicinal uses.

How to Use:

 INFUSED OIL: Milky oats are not typically infused into oil due to their water content. But oatstraw can be dried, then infused into oil for a skin-soothing, moisturizing option.

 TINCTURE: 1 part fresh milky oats to 2 parts 75% alcohol. Used for calming frazzled nerves, gently balancing the nervous system without heavy sedation, and deep nourishment.

 TEA: Steep 1 ounce dried oatstraw in 1 quart hot water for 4–8 hours. Longer infusions of oatstraw draw out nutritive minerals from the plant. Used for combating nervous exhaustion and fatigue and as a great source of minerals. For milky oats, lightly crush the fresh or frozen pods and steep 2 heaping tablespoons in 1 cup hot water, covered, for 10–15 minutes. Tea made with milky oats can provide an immediate calming effect in an acute setting as well as a boost of nutritive B vitamins and minerals.

 POULTICE AND COMPRESS: Moistened rolled oats can be applied as a poultice directly to rashes and irritation. A compress made with oatstraw tea can be used for similar support, but is less commonly used.

 BATH SOAK: Dried oats or oatstraw can be added to baths for itchy, inflamed skin or eczema.

General Safety:

TOPICAL USE: Very safe, even for infants.

INTERNAL USE: Safe as food and medicine. Extremely gentle. For pregnant and nursing women, oats are safe, nourishing, and recommended.

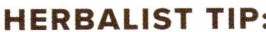

HERBALIST TIP:

You don't need a field of oats to be able to harvest enough milky oats and oatstraw to fill the average home apothecary. Even a 3' × 3' garden bed or plot can yield enough plants to give you a few bottles of tincture, plus oatstraw for baths and teas.

Mint

Mentha spp.

Perennial in zones 4–9 (variety dependent)

A hardy, fast-growing perennial herb with aromatic leaves, mint is prized for its refreshing flavor and digestive benefits.

Medicinal Properties:

TOPICAL: Cooling and analgesic. Anti-inflammatory; can relieve itching.

INTERNAL: Digestive aid, nausea relief, and mild pain relief. Helps reduce internal heat during fevers and hot weather. Its vapors open nasal passages, and its aroma can stimulate focus and clarity without overstimulation.

ENERGETIC: Cooling, drying.

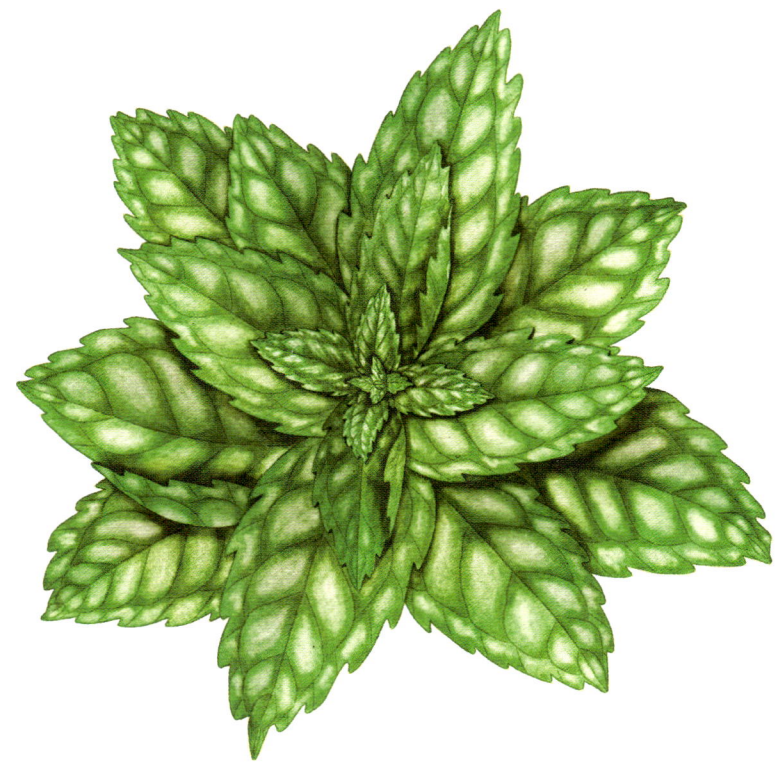

How to Grow:

 WHEN TO PLANT: Sow or transplant after the danger of frost has passed. In mild climates, start seeds indoors 6–8 weeks before last frost.

 GROWS BEST FROM: Seed, transplant, or propagation. Sow seeds on the soil surface and gently press in. Keep soil moist and warm for better germination. Seeds need light to germinate. Germination can take from 10–15 days. Direct sowing may be difficult with how tiny mint seeds are. Mint easily propagates in water or soil. Divide established clumps in spring or fall to transplant.

 SUN AND SOIL NEEDS: Full sun to partial shade. Needs more shade in hotter climates, specifically in the afternoon. Prefers fertile, well-draining soil with moderate, consistent moisture. Can tolerate growing in more shade than the average herb.

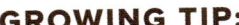

GROWING TIP:

Mint is famously vigorous. It spreads aggressively by underground runners and can quickly take over a garden bed. Many gardeners keep it in pots or contained areas to enjoy the fresh, cooling leaves without letting it dominate the herb patch.

 VARIETIES TO TRY: Peppermint, spearmint, Kentucky Colonel spearmint, chocolate mint, apple mint, orange mint, grapefruit mint, variegated pineapple mint, and Corsican mint.

 SPACING: Space plants 18–24" apart for vigorous spread. Mint will quickly fill in gaps, so this spacing gives each plant room to breathe without overcrowding. In containers, space one plant per 12–16" diameter pot for full, bushy growth. Use a deep pot (at least 10–12") to keep roots contained. Place a self-watering dish or base under pots to help avoid the spread of runners.

 BLOOM TIME: 60–90 days from seed to initial small harvest. Typically 90–100 days from seed to when plants are well-established. Produces flowers in the summer.

 HARVESTING TIPS: Begin harvesting leaves once plants are at least 8–12" tall. The best flavor and potency is just before plants start to flower. If you need usable leaves sooner, start mint from cuttings or divisions. You can harvest within 4–6 weeks instead of waiting 2–3 months from seed.

How to Use:

 INFUSED OIL: Infuse dried leaves into oils, salves, and balms for topical use. Serves as a cooling solution for muscles, a refreshing massage oil, or a lip balm flavor.

 TINCTURE: 1 part fresh herb to 2 parts 95% alcohol; tincture fresh to preserve the volatile oils. Provides concentrated relief for digestive upset and tension headaches.

 TEA: Steep 1–2 teaspoons dried leaves per 1 cup hot or cold water, covered, for 5–10 minutes. Or, steep 2–3 tablespoons fresh leaves (roughly 5–6 sprigs, lightly smashed) per 1 cup hot water, covered, for 5–10 minutes. Used for nausea relief, to reduce gas and bloating and stomach spasms, as a decongestant, for headache relief, and for stress reduction.

 POULTICE AND COMPRESS: Used in poultices to help with tension headaches (apply to temples), mild skin irritation, and bug bites. Cold compresses can be used to cool a fever, soothe sunburn, and calm headaches.

〱〱〱 **STEAM INHALATION:** Add a handful of fresh leaves, or 1 tablespoon dried leaves, to a bowl of hot water. Tent your head with a towel and inhale vapors for 5–10 minutes. Used as a decongestant and mental stimulant, and for headache and nausea relief.

⚠ General Safety:

TOPICAL USE: Well tolerated by most people, but volatile oils can irritate sensitive skin. Do not apply peppermint or spearmint oil directly to mucous membranes (such as in nose or mouth) or sensitive skin without dilution to avoid burning sensation.

INTERNAL USE: Generally safe in culinary and tea amounts for most adults and children. Peppermint tea may aggravate acid reflux, as it can relax the esophageal sphincter. Safe in moderate culinary tea amounts for pregnant and nursing women (it is often used for morning sickness), but always consult your doctor before use. Avoid strong peppermint oil on the face of infants and small children, due to the risk of menthol-related breathing difficulty.

HERBALIST TIP:

Peppermint is more stimulating for acute relief, while spearmint is gentler and works well for daily or children's use.

Motherwort

Leonurus cardiaca
Hardy perennial in zones 3–8

An upright branching plant with square stems in the mint family, motherwort features deeply lobed leaves and small pink or purple flowers in whorls along the stem. The word *cardiaca* in this herb's scientific name points to its role in soothing stress-related palpitations and anxiety.

Medicinal Properties:

TOPICAL: Mildly antimicrobial. Sometimes used in poultices, but not a primary topical herb.

INTERNAL: Nervine, bitter tonic, and emmenagogue. Supports heart and circulation. Used for anxiety, restlessness, palpitations, menstrual cramps, and menopause symptoms.

ENERGETIC: Cooling, drying.

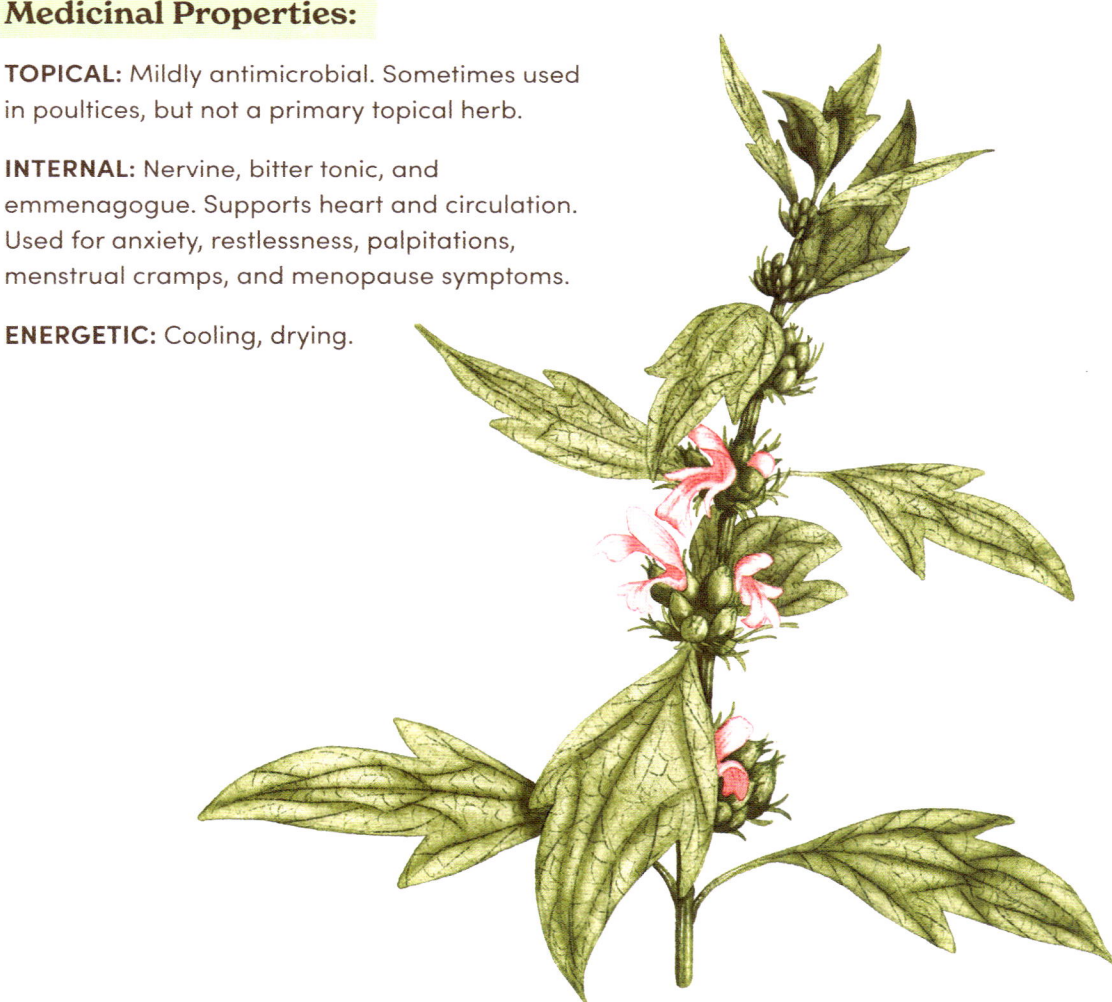

How to Grow:

 WHEN TO PLANT: Direct sow outdoors in fall in warmer winter regions, or in early spring in colder winter regions.

 GROWS BEST FROM: Seed. Motherwort self-seeds readily once established. Seeds are tiny, like mint seeds, and benefit from 2–3 weeks of cold stratification. Sow seeds on the surface of the soil and keep moist. Germination takes 2–3 weeks. Transplant after 4–6 weeks.

 SUN AND SOIL NEEDS: Full sun to partial shade. Tolerates a wide range of soils, but prefers moderately rich, well-drained soil.

 VARIETIES TO TRY: Common motherwort and Siberian motherwort.

 SPACING: Plants are tall and branching, so sow seeds 18–24" apart to give plenty of airflow. Can be grown in a larger container.

 BLOOM TIME: 100–120 days from seed to peak harvest of aerial parts (flowers, stems and leaves) when planted in the spring, or once plant breaks dormancy in spring if established in the fall.

 HARVESTING TIPS: Begin light harvests of aerial tops in 90–100 days after seeding, once plants reach about 2' tall. Collect aerial parts at first bloom, usually midsummer, at 100–120 days.

GOOD TO KNOW:

The name motherwort reflects this herb's traditional use in women's health. It can help ease menstrual cramps, and it can promote delayed menstruation and calm postpartum nerves and heart rate racing after childbirth.

How to Use:

 INFUSED OIL: Not typically made with this herb.

 TINCTURE: 1 part fresh herb to 2 parts 50–60% alcohol, or 1 part dried herb to 5 parts 40–50% alcohol. Used to reduce menstrual cramps, acute anxiety, and nervous heart palpitations. Can also induce menstruation with its emmenagogue properties.

 TEA: Steep 1–2 teaspoons dried herb per 1 cup hot water for 10 minutes. It is very bitter, so it is often blended with milder herbs (fresh motherwort is more bitter than dried, so it is not typically used for teas). Teas are not often used, but they can have similar beneficial properties as tinctures.

 POULTICE AND COMPRESS: Not commonly used with this herb.

 BATH SOAK: Steep ½–1 cup dried motherwort in 1 quart hot water for 20–30 minutes, then add to your bathwater for tension or menstrual cramp relief.

⚠ General Safety:

TOPICAL USE: Generally safe, though rarely used externally.

INTERNAL USE: Generally safe, but the bitterness can cause nausea in high doses. This herb may interact with thyroid or heart medications, such as digitalis or beta blockers. Not recommended during pregnancy, as it is an emmenagogue and a mild uterine stimulant that can encourage contractions.

HERBALIST TIP:

The bitterness of motherwort makes tincturing preferred over consuming this herb in a tea.

Mugwort

Artemisia vulgaris
Hardy perennial in zones 4–9

This tall, aromatic herb has deeply lobed, dark green leaves that are white and downy underneath and clusters of small greenish-yellow to greenish-white flowers.

Medicinal Properties:

TOPICAL: Supports healing of bruises, sore muscles, and joint pain.

INTERNAL: Bitter tonic, carminative, emmenagogue, and nervine. Used for poor appetite, sluggish digestion and lymph stagnation, menstrual irregularities, headaches, and mild anxiety. Can also encourage vivid dreams.

ENERGETIC: Cooling, drying.

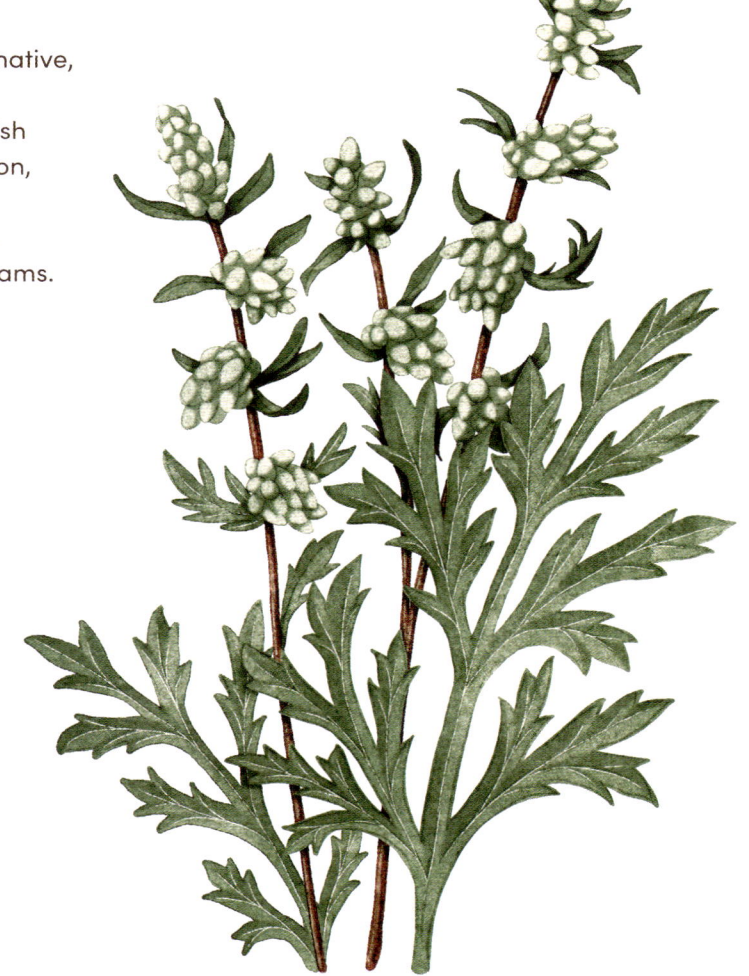

How to Grow:

 WHEN TO PLANT: Direct sow outdoors in spring after last frost, or start indoors 6–8 weeks before last frost.

 GROWS BEST FROM: Seed, root division, or cuttings (it spreads easily by rhizomes). The seeds are very small, almost like dust, and need light to germinate, so sow on the surface of the soil. Germination can take 14–21 days. Once seedlings have 2–3 sets of adult leaves, thin to one plant per pot and let grow for 4–6 more weeks before transplanting outside. To divide plants, simply dig up chunks of root systems and plant in a new spot.

 SUN AND SOIL NEEDS: Full sun to partial shade. Tolerates poor soils and drought once established.

 VARIETIES TO TRY: Common mugwort and California mugwort.

 SPACING: Space plants 24–36" apart to allow room for spreading plants. Mugwort plants can get 3–6' tall and 2–3' wide when conditions are right. Containing it to a planter or large pot can avoid that spread.

 BLOOM TIME: 90–100 days from initial sowing.

 HARVESTING TIPS: Peak harvest is best just before or at early flowering stage (mid to late summer) for medicinal use, 90–100 days.

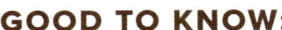

GOOD TO KNOW:

Mugwort has a long history in European, Asian, and Native American traditions as a dream herb because it can enhance vivid dreams when taken as a tea, smoked, or placed under pillows in a sachet. It was also called the "mother of herbs" in European folk medicine.

How to Use:

 INFUSED OIL: Dried herb can be infused for massage oils targeting aches, cramps, and cold joints.

 TINCTURE: 1 part fresh herb to 2 parts 50–60% alcohol, or 1 part dried herb to 5 parts 40–50% alcohol. Used as a bitter tonic to aid in sluggish digestion, as a mild nervine to ease anxiety, and as an emmenagogue to promote menstruation. Can also minimize headaches.

 TEA: Steep 1 teaspoon dried herb per 1 cup hot water for 10–15 minutes (fresh mugwort has a strong flavor and is not usually used for teas). Used for digestion, menstrual support, or dream work.

 POULTICE AND COMPRESS: Although not often used, crushed fresh leaves can be applied as a poultice to sore muscles or bruises. Compresses made with mugwort tea are not often used.

 General Safety:

TOPICAL USE: Safe in moderation. Essential oils may cause irritation in sensitive skin.

INTERNAL USE: Avoid in high doses because of potential neurotoxicity. Pregnant and nursing women should avoid internal use, as mugwort is a strong emmenagogue and may stimulate uterine contractions.

HERBALIST TIP:

Mugwort is best used as a ritual, digestive, and dream herb, not an everyday tonic. Think of it when you need warming stimulation, menstrual support, or to connect with the herbal traditions of ancestors.

Mullein

Verbascum thapsus
Biennial in zones 3–9

This classic lung remedy is known as "nature's Mucinex." A tall, fuzzy-leaved herb with bright yellow flowers, it lives its full life cycle in a 2-year timeframe.

Medicinal Properties:

TOPICAL: Mild support for skin wounds, rashes, and swelling. Mullein flower–infused oil can help with ear pain and infections.

INTERNAL: Respiratory support and helpful in both dry and productive coughs. Anti-inflammatory. Mild demulcent that can soothe inflamed gut lining and urinary tract.

ENERGETIC: Cooling, moistening.

HERBALIST TIP:

As a steward of nature, it's important to take invasive plants like mullein seriously, as they can take over an area. Grow it in a controlled space to best manage seed spread. In the second year of growth, remove flowering stalks to avoid widespread seed dispersal.

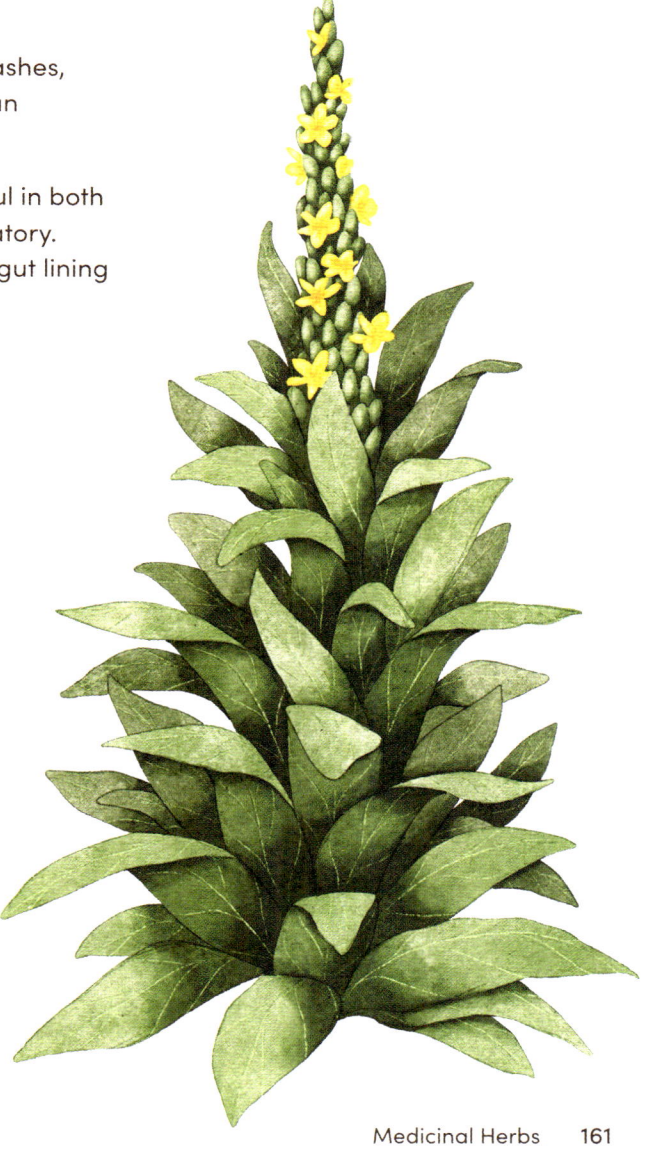

How to Grow:

 WHEN TO PLANT: Sow or transplant after the danger of frost has passed. In mild climates, start seeds indoors 6–8 weeks before last frost.

 GROWS BEST FROM: Seed. Mullein seeds are very tiny and need light to germinate, so press lightly into soil and keep moist. Cold stratifying mullein seeds can help improve germination. One mullein plant can produce thousands of seeds in its second year, which is what helps it become so invasive in many areas of the United States. This is also why you won't find many nurseries selling live transplants of mullein.

 SUN AND SOIL NEEDS: Full sun, 6–8 hours or more. Mullein will bloom better and has lower risk for fungal disease in full sun. Prefers well-draining, sandy soil and tolerates poor-quality growing conditions. Drought tolerant once established.

 VARIETIES TO TRY: Common mullein, Greek mullein, white mullein, and hybrid mullein.

 SPACING: Sow seeds at least 18–24" apart to allow proper airflow. The leaf spread of a second-year mullein plant can reach almost 36" if conditions are right, so allow the space. Plants will grow low to the ground the first year and send up a tall flower spike the second year that can reach up to 48" tall.

 BLOOM TIME: Mullein is a biennial and will only produce leaves in its first year of growth. After overwintering, the plant will produce more leaves in its second year and will send up a tall flower stalk. This will produce yellow flowers all along the stalk that will dry out and produce thousands of seeds. After this stage, the plant will die entirely.

 HARVESTING TIPS: From seed to first usable leaf harvest is between 3–4 months, and from seed to flower harvest is 12–18 months. If you intend to harvest the roots of the plant, you will want to harvest them in the first year of growth, as the plant's energy is focused in that part of the plant during that time. Harvest leaves in late spring through summer of the first year once they have matured but are still tender. Choose healthy green leaves free of spots or mildew. Don't take more than ⅓ of the leaves from a single plant at a time.

How to Use:

 INFUSED OIL: Oil infusions can be made with fresh mullein flowers. Let flowers wilt for a few hours to reduce moisture content and lower mold risk.

 TINCTURE: 1 part dried herb (leaves) to 5 parts 40–50% alcohol. Acts as an expectorant and demulcent.

 TEA: Steep 2–3 teaspoons dried flowers, or ¼ cup fresh leaves/flowers, per 1 cup hot water, covered, for 5–10 minutes. Carefully strain through a fine-mesh sieve or cheesecloth to remove the leaves' tiny hairs to prevent throat irritation. Used as a gentle and soothing expectorant to loosen mucus in the lungs or as a mild diuretic to cleanse and soothe the urinary tract.

 POULTICE AND COMPRESS: Used in poultices for boils, abscesses, and skin infections. Compresses can be used on the chest for coughs and congestion.

 STEAM INHALATION: Add a handful of fresh leaves, or 2–3 tablespoons dried leaves, to a bowl of hot water. Tent your head with a towel and inhale vapors for 5–10 minutes to help open airways and calm dry, hacking coughs or lingering bronchial irritation.

⚠ General Safety:

TOPICAL USE: Generally safe for topical use. The fine hairs on the leaves of mullein may irritate sensitive skin, so strain any oils or infusions through a fine-mesh sieve or cheesecloth.

INTERNAL USE: Mullein leaf tea is generally seen as safe for pregnant or nursing women, but high medicinal doses should be avoided.

GOOD TO KNOW:

Mullein has a few nicknames, such as torch plant and cowboy toilet paper. It's called "torch plant" because the tall stalks of dried seed heads that form in its second year of growth can be covered in wax or tallow and burned as torches. Mullein's soft leaves are a weary outdoor traveler's convenient toilet paper. (Mullein has an invasive nature and is often found in the wild.)

Nasturtium

Tropaeolum majus
Annual

These trailing or bushy plants have rounded shield-like leaves and showy, edible flowers in shades of red, orange, and yellow. Nasturtium is a vibrant edible flower in the garden, known for its peppery leaf and flower taste.

Medicinal Properties:

TOPICAL: Antimicrobial that treats bug bites and skin eruptions.

INTERNAL: Antimicrobial and expectorant. Circulatory stimulant. Relieves coughs and colds. Used as a "natural antibiotic" due to its spicy mustard compounds.

ENERGETIC: Warming, slightly drying.

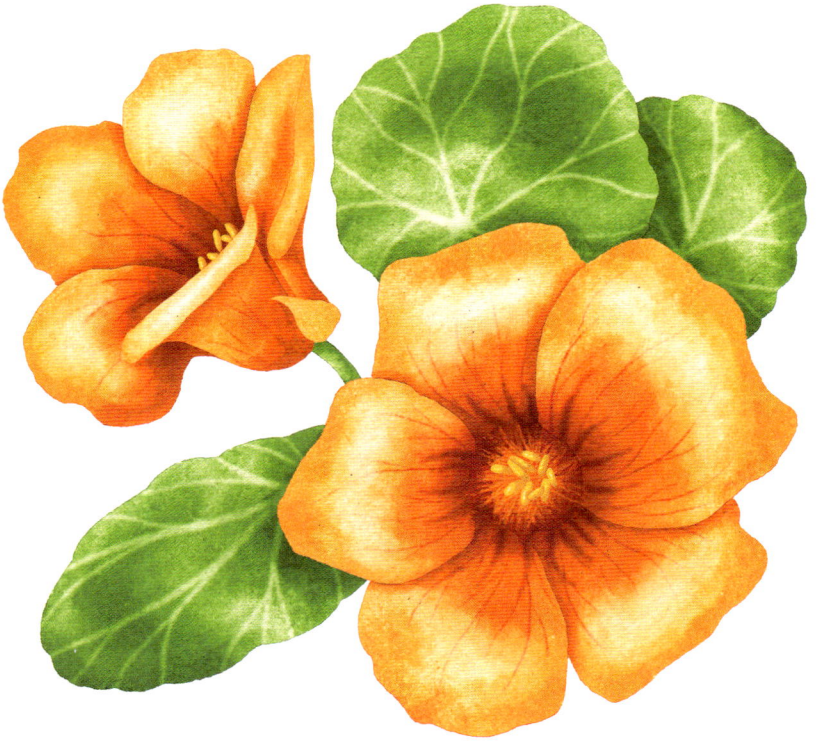

How to Grow:

 WHEN TO PLANT: Direct sow outdoors after last frost. Seeds germinate best in soil that has warmed to 55–65°F. Does not transplant well and grows best in cooler weather in transitional seasons.

 GROWS BEST FROM: Seed. Seeds are large, easy to handle, and quick to sprout. Press seeds ¼" into the soil and keep moist. Germination takes 7–14 days.

 SUN AND SOIL NEEDS: Full sun to partial shade. Prefers poor-to-average, well-drained soil. Rich soil produces lush leaves but fewer flowers. In hotter climates, plant nasturtium where it can get more shade to extend the life of the plant.

 VARIETIES TO TRY: Jewel Mix, Empress of India, and trailing varieties.

 SPACING: Sow seeds 8–12" apart for bush types. Trailing varieties need more room. Plant along edges of pathways or garden beds to allow plants to trail over the edges.

 BLOOM TIME: Leaves are ready 4–6 weeks after sowing. Flowers begin 8–10 weeks from seeding and continue all summer.

 HARVESTING TIPS: Harvest leaves once the plant has established, at 4–6 weeks. Flowers can be picked once they start to bloom a few weeks later. Harvest green seed pods for "capers" 10–12 weeks after seeding.

GOOD TO KNOW:

Nasturtium leaves, flowers, and seed pods are all edible. The leaves add a peppery flavor to salads, the flowers make vibrant garnishes, and the green seed pods are known as the "poor man's caper" when pickled. The leaves, flowers, and green pods can be infused into apple cider vinegar for 2–4 weeks to make a peppery, vibrant, and medicinal addition to marinades or vinaigrettes.

How to Use:

 INFUSED OIL: Leaves and flowers can be infused in oil for antimicrobial skin use.

 TINCTURE: 1 part fresh leaves to 2 parts 50–60% alcohol. Used for antimicrobial respiratory or urinary support.

 TEA: Briefly steep 1 teaspoon fresh leaves/flowers per 1 cup hot water. Nasturtium has a pungent, spicy mustard flavor, so is best when lightly brewed with other, sweeter herbs. Used for clearing the lungs, loosening mucus, and urinary tract infections.

 POULTICE AND COMPRESS: Crushed fresh leaves can be used as a poultice on insect stings, small cuts, or skin eruptions. A compress made with nasturtium tea can have similar benefits, but is less effective than a poultice.

⚠ General Safety:

TOPICAL USE: Generally safe. May sting slightly on broken skin due to mustard compounds.

INTERNAL USE: Safe in culinary amounts. Large doses may cause stomach upset. Pregnant and nursing women should avoid concentrated medicinal doses as they can cause mild uterine stimulant activity.

HERBALIST TIP:

Nasturtium is an easy-to-grow multipurpose plant. It beautifies the garden, attracts pollinators, and provides both food and medicine. For the best flower production, don't overfertilize. For a more peppery flavor and stronger overall medicinal potency, allow the plant to sustain some stressful conditions (less watering, poor soil) to help increase the concentration of those properties.

Oregano

Origanum vulgare
Perennial in zones 5–10

This hardy, aromatic perennial herb has small green leaves and clusters of tiny purple-pink flowers that bloom in the summer. A staple in Mediterranean cooking, oregano is also a potent medicinal plant known for its antimicrobial, respiratory, and digestive benefits.

Medicinal Properties:

TOPICAL: Strong antibacterial and antifungal. Good for wound care and skin infections.

INTERNAL: Supports digestion and reduces bloating and gas. Relieves coughs and congestion. Natural antimicrobial against colds and flu. Can help cleanse the urinary tract and reduce fluid retention.

ENERGETIC: Warming, drying.

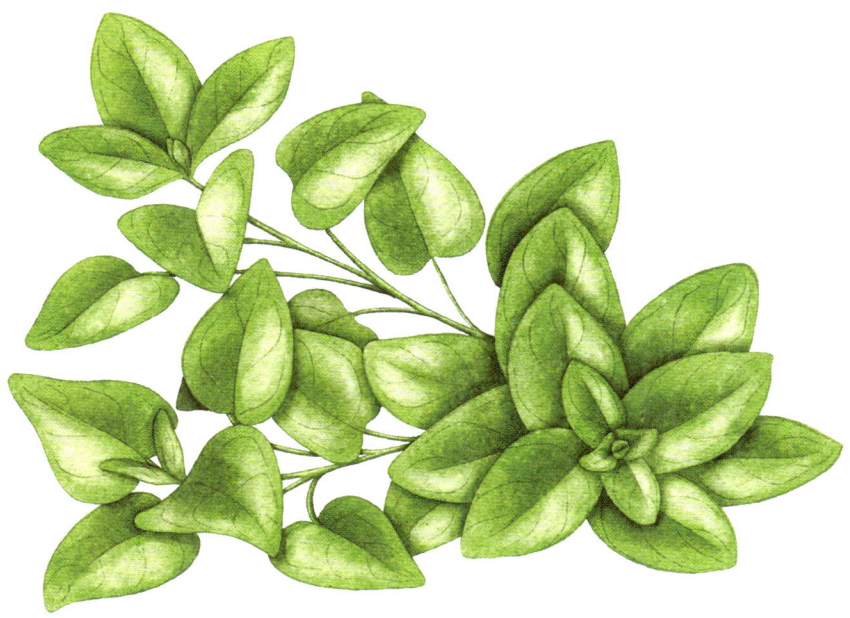

How to Grow:

 WHEN TO PLANT: Start seeds indoors 6–10 weeks before last frost, or direct sow outdoors after danger of frost has passed. Transplants are the easiest options for beginners.

 GROWS BEST FROM: Transplant, root division, or cuttings—although starting from seed is not impossible. Seeds can be slow to germinate (7–21 days). To divide the roots, you can dig up anytime in the active growing season and replant elsewhere to get more plants. Cuttings can be rooted easily in water and replanted into soil.

 SUN AND SOIL NEEDS: Full sun, 6–8 hours or more, and well-draining soil. Drought tolerant once established, but flavor is stronger in lean, slightly dry soil. Oregano thrives in Mediterranean conditions, with less frequent deep waterings and very loose soil that is able to dry out between waterings.

 VARIETIES TO TRY: Greek oregano, Italian oregano, Syrian oregano, and golden oregano.

 SPACING: Space plants 12–18" apart to allow for airflow, prevent mildew, and provide space for spreading. Some oregano can grow more bushy, but others will trail over the edges of garden beds and containers. Container friendly.

 BLOOM TIME: Typically 80–90 days from seed to harvest, or earlier if planted from cuttings or transplant.

 HARVESTING TIPS: Begin lightly harvesting once plants are 6" tall. Snip sprigs just before flowering for best flavor and medicinal potency.

GROWING TIP:

Oregano can spread aggressively in the garden and is best planted where it has room, or in containers to control growth. Bees love the flowers, making oregano both a medicinal herb and pollinator-friendly plant.

How to Use:

 INFUSED OIL: Dried leaves can be infused into oil for antimicrobial salves or chest rubs.

 TINCTURE: 1 part fresh herb to 2 parts 50–60% alcohol or 1 part dried herb to 5 parts 40% alcohol. Used for digestive or immune support.

 TEA: Steep 1 teaspoon dried leaves, or 1–2 tablespoons fresh leaves, per 1 cup hot water, covered, for 10–15 minutes. Used to numb a sore throat, shorten cold and flu duration, and support sluggish digestion.

 POULTICE AND COMPRESS: Crushed fresh leaves can be applied as a poultice to skin for infection, wounds, or fungal issues. A hot or cold compress made with oregano tea can be used to provide similar benefits.

SSS STEAM INHALATION: Add a handful of fresh leaves, or 2–3 tablespoons dried leaves, to a bowl of hot water. Tent your head with a towel and inhale vapors for 5–10 minutes to address respiratory congestion.

⚠ General Safety:

TOPICAL USE: Always dilute essential oil heavily in a carrier oil. Undiluted oil can burn skin. Infused oils are gentler and safer.

INTERNAL USE: Safe in culinary and tea amounts. Strong tinctures should be used only for the short term. Oregano can be harsh on the gut microbiome, so avoid extended internal use. Avoid high doses when on anticoagulant medications. For pregnant and nursing women, culinary use is safe, but medicinal extracts in high amounts should be avoided without professional guidance.

HERBALIST TIP:

Oregano tea combined with thyme makes a powerful respiratory tonic, soothing coughs and easing chest congestion while delivering strong antimicrobial benefits.

Passion Vine

Passiflora incarnata

Perennial in zones 6–10 (variety dependent)

This perennial climbing vine with delicate tendrils, deeply lobed leaves, and streaming purple and white flowers may produce maypops, or passion fruit. It is well known for its sedative and nervine properties.

Medicinal Properties:

TOPICAL: Not commonly used externally.

INTERNAL: Mild antispasmodic. Nervine that calms nervous system and mood, acts as a sleep aid, and soothes mood swings and irritability.

ENERGETIC: Cooling, slightly drying.

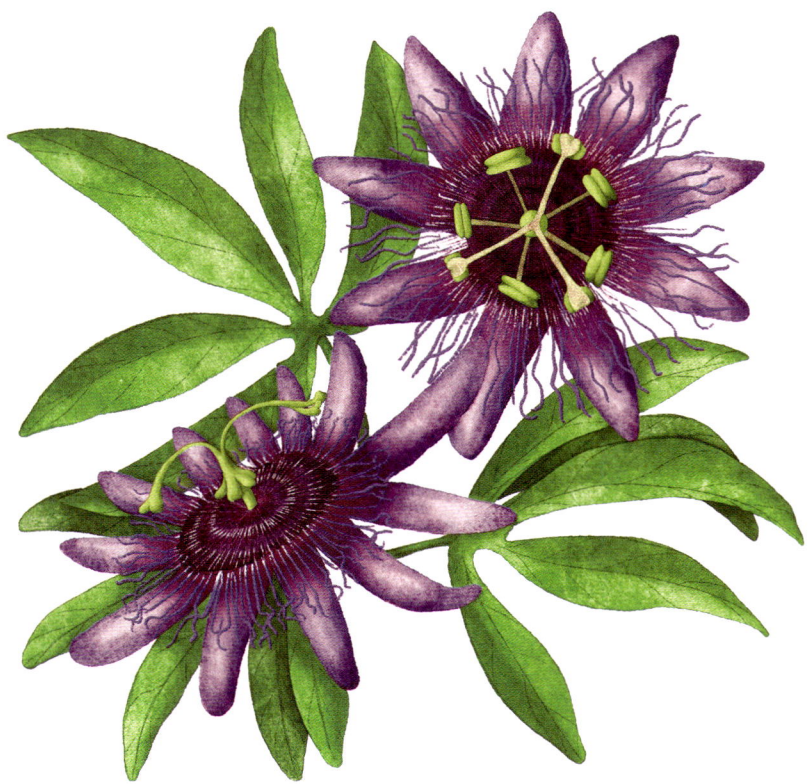

How to Grow:

 WHEN TO PLANT: Plant outdoors once soil temps are consistently above 60°F.

 GROWS BEST FROM: Seed, root division, or cuttings. Nick the seed coat, soak seeds overnight, and use heat mats indoors to speed germination. Can take up to 2–8 weeks to germinate. To divide the roots, take a clump of roots from the main plant in early spring and replant elsewhere. In late spring/early summer, take 4–6" sections, remove lower leaves, dip in rooting hormone, and place in moist soil or water until roots form.

 SUN AND SOIL NEEDS: Full sun to partial shade. Moderately fertile, well-draining soil is preferred, but this plant can tolerate some poorer soil conditions once established.

 VARIETIES TO TRY: Maypop, purple passion fruit, and yellow passion fruit.

 SPACING: Passion vine is an aggressive plant that can take over any structure nearby. Only 1 plant per 15–20' is necessary! Passion vine can grow as tall as the structure it grows on. Plant live plants along sturdy fences or trellis structures and be ready for more young plants to pop up via the root system as the season progresses in warmer climates.

 BLOOM TIME: From seed, harvestable material usually appears by the second growing season. Root division plants may take off enough within one active growing season.

 HARVESTING TIPS: Harvest fresh flowers in mid to late summer when they are fully open but not beginning to wilt. Choose young, tender to mid-mature leaves and harvest at any time during the active growing season. Avoid taking more than ⅓ of the plant while it's still young.

GOOD TO KNOW:

The passionflower variety *Passiflora incarnata* is the only host plant in the southwestern United States that the Gulf fritillary butterfly can feed off of. The flowers of this herb can turn into a round fruit, called a "maypop," that starts out green and turns yellow when ripe. It has a sweet and tart pulp that can be eaten fresh or used in drinks.

How to Use:

 INFUSED OIL: Not typically made with this herb.

 TINCTURE: 1 part fresh flowers and leaves to 2 parts 95% alcohol, or 1 part dried flowers and leaves to 5 parts 40–50% alcohol. Preparations made with flowers are less potent, but do still provide similar benefits as the leaves, such as promoting sleep onset, improving quality of sleep, reducing stress and circular thinking, and reducing the intensity of tension headaches.

 TEA: Steep 1–2 teaspoons dried leaves or flowers, or 2–3 tablespoons fresh leaves or flowers, per 1 cup hot water for 10–15 minutes. Fresh leaves have a more bitter, grassy flavor that can be covered with lemon or sweetener. Dried leaves are less pungent. Used to reduce stress and circular thinking and to promote restful sleep and easier sleep onset.

 POULTICE AND COMPRESS: Poultices and compresses can be applied for bruises or inflammation, but are less commonly used.

⚠ General Safety:

TOPICAL USE: Generally safe, though rarely used externally.

INTERNAL USE: Passion vine is generally gentle and well tolerated, but it can enhance the effects of sedatives or medications for sleep/anxiety. Always use in moderation and consult with a healthcare provider if combining with pharmaceuticals. Avoid use during pregnancy, as it can stimulate uterine contractions. Nursing mothers should consult with their doctors about use and monitor infants for drowsiness.

HERBALIST TIP:

Many herbalists prefer to tincture flowers and leaves together for a balanced nervine effect. If only using flowers, you can use the same ratios, but flowers tend to be lighter, so pack them well into your jars for tincturing.

Plantain Leaf

Plantago major, Plantago lanceolata
Perennial in zones 3–9

A highly common and humble wild edible herb, often called "nature's bandage." It is powerfully soothing and healing, and primarily used as a quick, topical remedy for stings, bites, and minor cuts due to its strong drawing and soothing properties.

Medicinal Properties:

TOPICAL: Soothes insect bites, stings, burns, rashes, cuts, and minor wounds. Known as a "drawing" herb that can help pull out splinters, toxins, or infections.

INTERNAL: Acts as a demulcent, coating and soothing mucous membranes in the throat, lungs, stomach, and intestines. Mild astringent. Used for coughs, sore throats, ulcers, gastritis, and urinary irritation. The seeds of plantain are used as a fiber supplement that has soothing mucilage to help aid in relieving constipation and supporting better digestion.

ENERGETIC: Cooling, moistening.

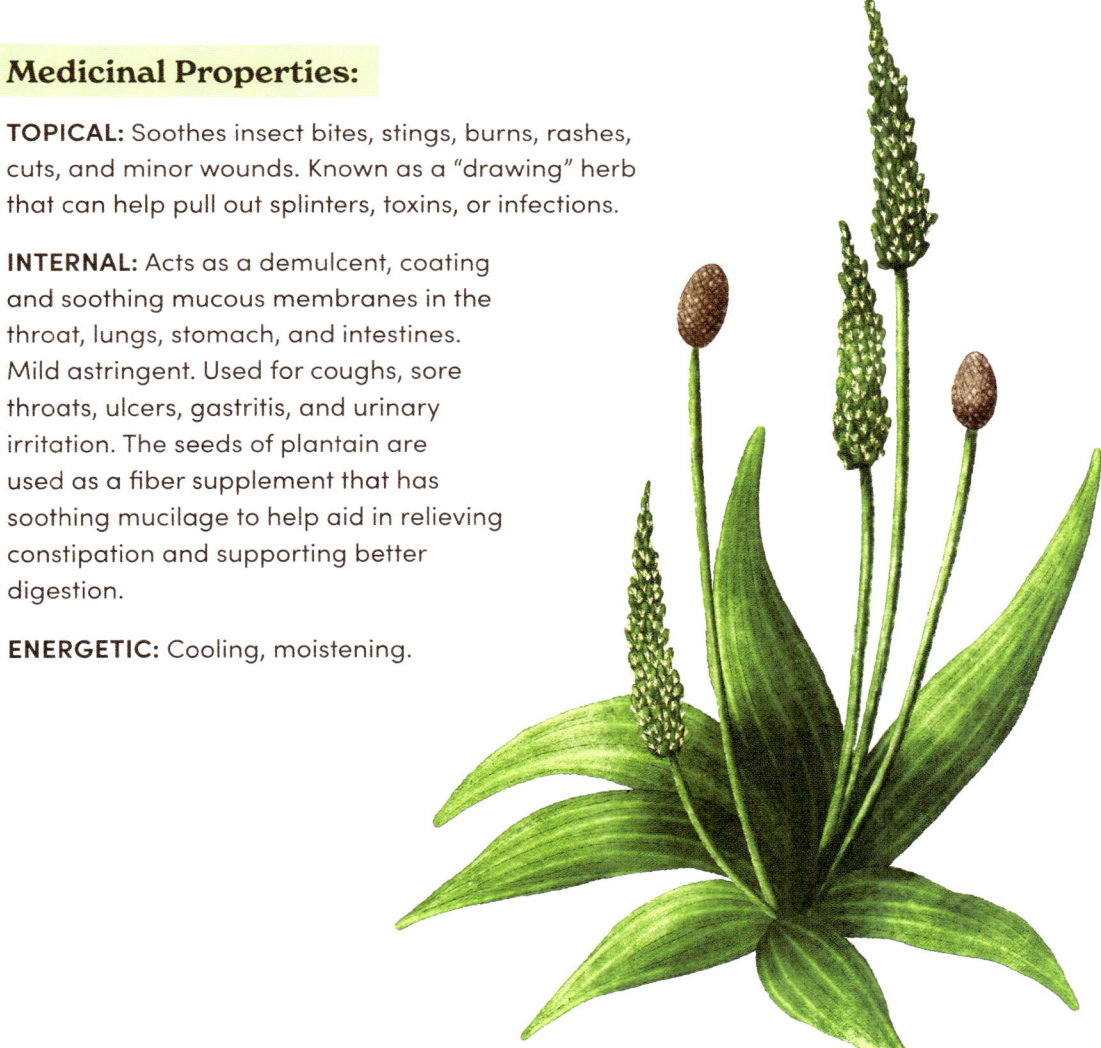

How to Grow:

 WHEN TO PLANT: Sow seeds outdoors in early spring or fall. Plantain thrives in disturbed soil and will self-seed if allowed to flower.

 GROWS BEST FROM: Seed or root division. Seeds need light to germinate. Surface sow and keep moist. Root divisions from mature plants transplant easily.

 SUN AND SOIL NEEDS: Full sun to partial shade. Adaptable to most soils, but prefers moist, well-draining ground. Tolerates compacted soils, making it common in paths and lawns.

 VARIETIES TO TRY: Broadleaf plantain and narrowleaf, or ribwort plantain.

 SPACING: Space plants 8–12" apart. Plantain forms low rosettes and spreads outward. Eventually, a spike will form that produces seeds, but overall this plant acts more like a ground cover.

 BLOOM TIME: Typically 6–8 weeks from seed to harvest. Plantain plants pop up in the wild in late spring to early summer in the lower half of North America.

 HARVESTING TIPS: Pick fresh young leaves anytime for topical use or for drying.

GROWING TIP:

Plantain grows abundantly in the wild. In suburban or landscaped areas, it is seen as a weed, as it pops up randomly, so be careful when foraging in areas that may be regularly sprayed with herbicides.

How to Use:

 INFUSED OIL: Fresh or dried leaves can be infused for salves that soothe skin, rashes, and bug bites.

 TINCTURE: Not typically made with this herb.

 TEA: Steep 1–2 teaspoons dried leaves, or 1–2 tablespoons fresh leaves, per 1 cup hot water, covered, for 10–15 minutes. Use to soothe the digestive tract and a dry, irritated throat as an internal wound healer. Can also be used as a mild expectorant and diuretic.

 POULTICE AND COMPRESS: Crushed fresh leaves can be applied as a poultice directly to bites, stings, or cuts. Dried leaves can be rehydrated for compresses. Plantain is often called "nature's bandage" for this reason. (The fresh leaf can even be chewed and applied directly as a spit poultice in emergencies for bee stings or cuts.)

 General Safety:

TOPICAL USE: Very safe for all ages. Minimal risk.

INTERNAL USE: Generally safe in tea or food amounts. High doses may have mild laxative effects due to seed mucilage. Considered safe in moderate culinary or tea use for pregnant and nursing women.

HERBALIST TIP:

Plantain is especially helpful for "hot and dry" conditions, like dry coughs, irritated throat, or inflamed skin. Pair it with other demulcents like marshmallow root for deeper internal soothing. The seeds of this herb's seed stalks can be used as a fiber supplement to ease constipation as well.

Roselle Hibiscus

Hibiscus sabdariffa
Annual

This heat-loving, drought-tolerant tropical plant, also known as sorrel, produces beautiful flowers that turn into edible calyxes used for teas and natural dye.

Medicinal Properties:

TOPICAL: Used as a toner to tighten and soothe skin, in compresses for sunburns, and as a hair rinse for scalp health.

INTERNAL: Rich in vitamin C antioxidants. Cools body heat, treats fever, supports lowering of blood pressure, and hydrates. Digestive stimulant, astringent (dries mucus), and diuretic.

ENERGETIC: Cooling, drying.

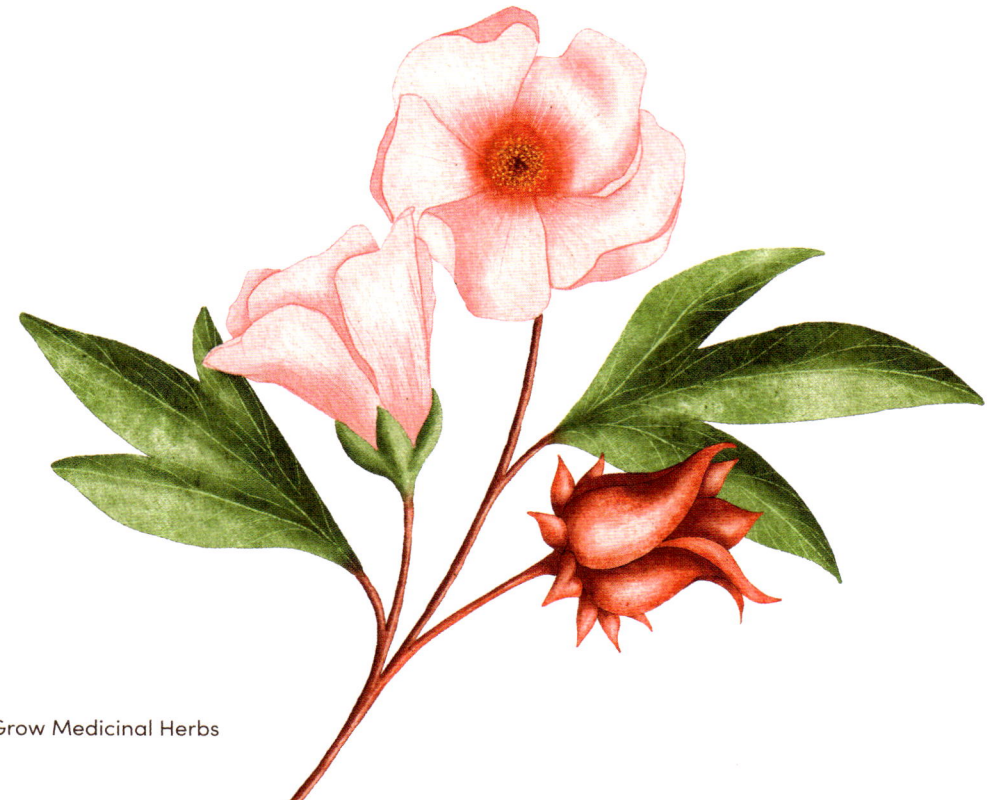

How to Grow:

 WHEN TO PLANT: Start indoors (using a heat mat) 6–8 weeks before transplanting into soil once temps have warmed above 70°F. Or, direct sow once soil temps are warmer, well after the last frost—more like early summertime.

 GROWS BEST FROM: Seed or transplant. Plant seeds ¼" deep. Lightly cover with soil or compost and keep moist, but not waterlogged.

 SUN AND SOIL NEEDS: Full sun—8 hours or more per day is ideal. Roselle loves heat! Avoid shade for this plant, which may lead to poor calyx formation. Once established, roselle can tolerate heat and some drought because of sturdy taproots.

 VARIETIES TO TRY: Thai red roselle, early roselle, green Senegalese roselle, and Burmese roselle.

 SPACING: Space plants 3–4' apart. Roselle plants can get up to 5–7' tall and are fairly wide thanks to branching at the top. Once plants are 12" tall, cut off the top third of the plant to encourage more branching. This creates a more manageable, bushy plant with a lot of branches to produce calyx on.

 BLOOM TIME: 90–120 days after transplanting. Add 2–3 weeks to this timeline if direct sowing.

 HARVESTING TIPS: Harvest calyxes after the flower petals fall off from the blooms, but before the seed pod inside becomes hard. The calyx should be plump, red, and tender, not woody.

GROWING TIP:

Roselle hibiscus plants are daylength sensitive, which means they will not begin to flower and create calyxes (the fleshy structures left after flowers have faded) until the days get shorter in the fall, when the amount of daylight falls below 12–13 hours. If started too early in the spring, the shorter days can trigger early calyx production. The calyx can be eaten fresh and used for jams, sauces, or teas.

How to Use:

 INFUSED OIL: Not typically made with this herb.

 TINCTURE: 1 part dried calyxes to 5 parts 40% alcohol to support lowering blood pressure, calm inflammation, and support the circulatory system.

 TEA: Steep 2–3 dried calyxes per 1 cup hot water for 8–10 minutes for a tea that is cooling, hydrating, stimulating, and tangy in flavor.

 POULTICE AND COMPRESS: Not typically used as a poultice or compress.

 General Safety:

TOPICAL USE: Well tolerated by most people. Can stain clothing or skin.

INTERNAL USE: Not recommended for pregnant or nursing mothers. Can lower blood pressure and blood sugar, which can be an issue for some people. Herbs with diuretic properties can cause dehydration if you don't maintain water intake alongside them. Can slow iron absorption if overconsumed.

HERBALIST TIP:

Roselle blends well with herbs like ginger and cinnamon. It can also be used as a facial toner or hair rinse to tone skin and stimulate the scalp for hair health.

Rosemary

Salvia rosmarinus
Perennial in zones 7–10

A woody, evergreen Mediterranean shrub with needle-shaped, aromatic leaves and pale blue flowers that bloom in the summer, rosemary is treasured as both a culinary herb and a powerful medicinal ally.

Medicinal Properties:

TOPICAL: Stimulates circulation, relieves sore muscles, and supports scalp health.

INTERNAL: Improves memory and concentration, supports healthy digestion, and stimulates circulation. Can gently improve mood and reduce headache symptoms.

ENERGETIC: Warming, drying.

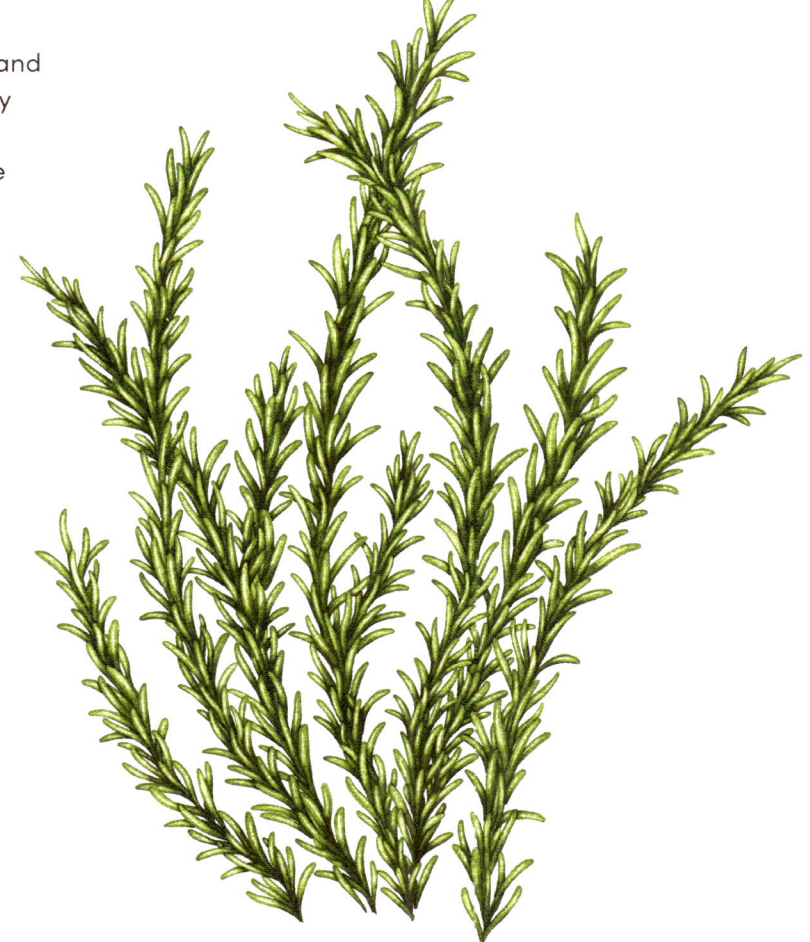

How to Grow:

 WHEN TO PLANT: Transplants can be planted in fall or spring outside in mild winter climates or in the spring after the threat of frost has passed in colder climates.

 GROWS BEST FROM: Transplant or rooted cuttings. Seeds are slow and sometimes finicky to germinate. Softwood cuttings root readily in water or moist soil. Transplants can give you a big head start in growing, because woody herbs can grow slowly.

 SUN AND SOIL NEEDS: Full sun, 6–8 hours or more. Much like lavender, rosemary prefers well-draining sandy or rocky soil. Rosemary dislikes "wet feet," meaning it doesn't like its roots to remain wet, so avoid watering it frequently. In fact, some purposeful neglect can really help your rosemary thrive!

 VARIETIES TO TRY: Arp, Tuscan Blue, *Prostratus* (creeping rosemary), and Blue Spires.

 SPACING: Space plants 18–24" apart in rows or clusters. Rosemary grows into a woody shrub over time, so it needs room for airflow and branching. Large varieties (like the upright shrub–form types, Arp or Tuscan Blue) need 24–36" between plants so they can reach their full size. Creeping varieties can spread 2–3' across, so give them space to cascade properly. In containers, allow only one plant per 12–16" container.

 BLOOM TIME: Typically 6–12 months from seed to even a small harvest. From cuttings, you can begin light harvesting within 3–6 months.

 HARVESTING TIPS: Harvest leaves anytime once the plant is established (usually after the first season). For peak flavor and oil content, harvest just before flowering.

GOOD TO KNOW:

Rosemary has antioxidant and antimicrobial properties, giving it a role in preserving food. Rosemary oil contains compounds that slow down lipid oxidation (the process that makes oils and fats go rancid). This is why it is used in commercial meat, deli meat, and poultry to slow fat spoilage and maintain fresh color.

How to Use:

 INFUSED OIL: Rosemary can be infused for muscle rubs, chest rubs, or scalp oils.

 TINCTURE: 1 part fresh herb to 2 parts 95% alcohol, or 1 part dried herb to 5 parts 40% alcohol. Used for cognitive support and improving mood, stimulating circulation, and reducing headache symptoms.

 TEA: Steep 1 teaspoon dried leaves, or 1–2 tablespoons fresh leaves, per 1 cup hot water, covered, for 10–15 minutes. Used for increasing memory and focus, improving digestion, and improving circulation.

 POULTICE AND COMPRESS: A warm rosemary compress can help soothe muscle soreness and pain or improve circulation in cold extremities. Poultices are not commonly used because of the potential for skin irritation.

))) **STEAM INHALATION:** Add a handful of fresh needles, or 2–3 tablespoons dried needles, to a bowl of hot water. Tent your head with a towel and inhale vapors for 5–10 minutes to clear sinuses and invigorate the mind.

⚠ General Safety:

TOPICAL USE: Generally safe, but essential oil is very strong, so always dilute it.

INTERNAL USE: Avoid very high doses because it can cause stomach upset. Culinary use is safe, but avoid medicinal strength doses in pregnant or nursing mothers.

HERBALIST TIP:

Rosemary has a strong connection to the head and circulatory system, which is why it shows up in traditional memory formulas. Rosemary tea or even just a sprig in hot water can act as a gentle pick-me-up when you're mentally foggy. It stimulates both mind and circulation without the jitteriness of caffeine.

Roses and Rose Hips

Rosa spp.
Perennial in zones 5–10

A beloved ornamental and medicinal plant, roses are valued for their fragrant petals and vitamin-rich fruits (called rose hips). Beyond their beauty, roses have a long history in folk medicine for their cooling, calming, and emotionally uplifting properties.

Medicinal Properties:

TOPICAL: Rose petals can soothe inflamed or irritated skin, such as for burns, rashes, acne, and mature skin.

INTERNAL: Rose petals and hips act as a mild nervine that can help uplift the heart and ease grief and anxiety. They can also reduce inflammation in the digestive tract, calm sore throats, support immunity, and improve circulatory sluggishness and lymph stagnation.

ENERGETIC: Cooling, moistening.

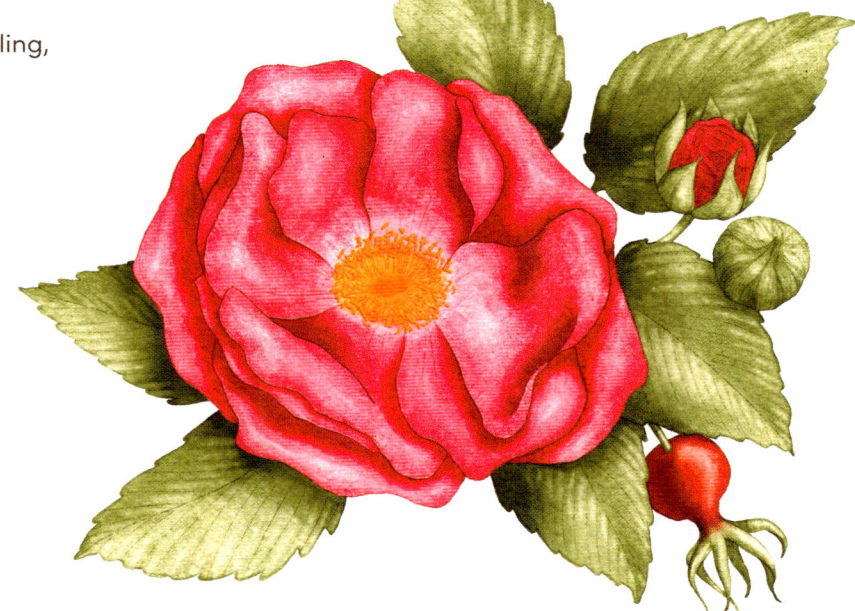

How to Grow:

 WHEN TO PLANT: Bare roots (dormant plants without leaves) are best planted in late winter to very early spring. In warm southern regions, you can often transplant bare roots as early as January or February. In colder regions, wait to transplant bare roots until the soil is workable and not frozen, usually in March or April. For potted, actively growing roses, plant after the last frost has passed.

 GROWS BEST FROM: Transplant, bare roots, or stem cuttings. Roses from seed are slow and variable. To make a cutting (propagation), take a 4–6" piece of stem from healthy, nonflowering growth, remove the lower leaves, and dip the cut end in rooting hormone. Plant this cutting in moist, well-draining soil or sand; cover to maintain consistent humidity; and keep warm until roots form in 3–6 weeks, then transplant outside after danger of frost has passed.

 SUN AND SOIL NEEDS: Full sun, 6–8 hours or more, is needed for best blooming and lower risk of fungal issues. Rich, well-draining soil with regular compost additions is best for good blooms and plant health.

 VARIETIES TO TRY: Damask rose, Apothecary rose, *Rosa rugosa*, and wild roses.

 SPACING: Space plants 2–4' apart, depending on growth habit. More spacing is best for vining varieties that can easily cover a trellis and more. Airflow is very important for roses, and fungal issues are a big risk for most varieties. Some varieties are bred for better resistance to these issues. Larger-container friendly, depending on variety.

 BLOOM TIME: Live rose plants may bloom within 6–8 weeks of transplanting. Bare root roses need 10–12 weeks after planting before producing their first flush of blooms. Rose hips will start to mature 6–8 weeks after the petals have dropped (for rose hip–producing varieties).

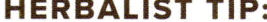

HERBALIST TIP:

Always choose fragrant, old-fashioned, or wild rose varieties for herbal use, as they have higher concentrations of volatile oils and beneficial compounds. Dry rose petals whole and crush them just before tea making to preserve nutrients. You can also steep fresh petals in distilled water for 30 minutes and mix with 1 teaspoon of witch hazel to make a soothing facial toner that keeps for short periods in the fridge.

HARVESTING TIPS: Harvest petals early in the morning when blooms are just opening for peak fragrance and oil content. Harvest rose hips in late summer through fall, after the flowers fade and the hips are plump, firm, and richly colored (usually a bright red/orange). Wait until after the first light frost if you want sweeter hips. To encourage rose hip production, let some blooms remain on the plant after peak flowering so the hips can set and mature.

How to Use:

 INFUSED OIL: Petals can be infused in a light carrier oil for skin care, balms, and massage oils.

 TINCTURE: 1 part fresh petals to 2 parts 80–95% alcohol, or 1 part dried petals to 5 parts 40% alcohol. Tinctures concentrate the cooling properties of roses, but this is not a typical use for extracting the medicinal properties of this herb.

 TEA: Steep 1–2 teaspoons dried petals, or ¼ cup fresh petals, per 1 cup hot water for 10–15 minutes. Calming, cooling, and heart soothing. For rose hips, steep 1 teaspoon crushed, dried rose hips, or 2–3 fresh sliced large hips, per 1 cup hot water, covered, for 10–15 minutes. Teas made with

fresh plant parts extract the highest amount of vitamin C, but be sure to strain this infusion well as fresh rose hips contain tiny, irritating hairs.

 POULTICE AND COMPRESS: Crushed fresh petals can be infused into warm compresses for irritated eyes, burns, or inflamed skin. Although less often used, a poultice of crushed rose petals with a small amount of water can be applied to the skin for similar benefits as a compress.

 General Safety:

TOPICAL USE: Well tolerated.

INTERNAL USE: Safe for most people in tea or culinary doses. Rose hips may interact with blood-thinning medications. Generally considered safe for pregnant and nursing women in tea and culinary amounts.

GROWING TIP:

Rose hips are the fruit of the rose plant. After the rose flower is pollinated and the petals fall away, the base of the flower swells and develops into a small berry-type structure. Not all rose varieties produce hips.

Sage

Salvia officinalis
Perennial in zones 4–9

A woody, aromatic perennial herb with soft, gray-green leaves and purple-blue flowers that bloom in the summer, sage has long been valued as a culinary seasoning and medicinal plant for aiding memory, digestion, sweat regulation, cold and flu support, and sore throats.

Medicinal Properties:

TOPICAL: Antimicrobial and astringent. Treats sore throats, gum inflammation, minor wounds, and skin infections.

INTERNAL: Carminative digestive support (relieves bloating, gas, and sluggish digestion). Reduces excessive sweating and hot flashes. Nootropic (supports cognition, focus, and memory), antifungal, antiviral, and antimicrobial.

ENERGETIC: Warming, drying.

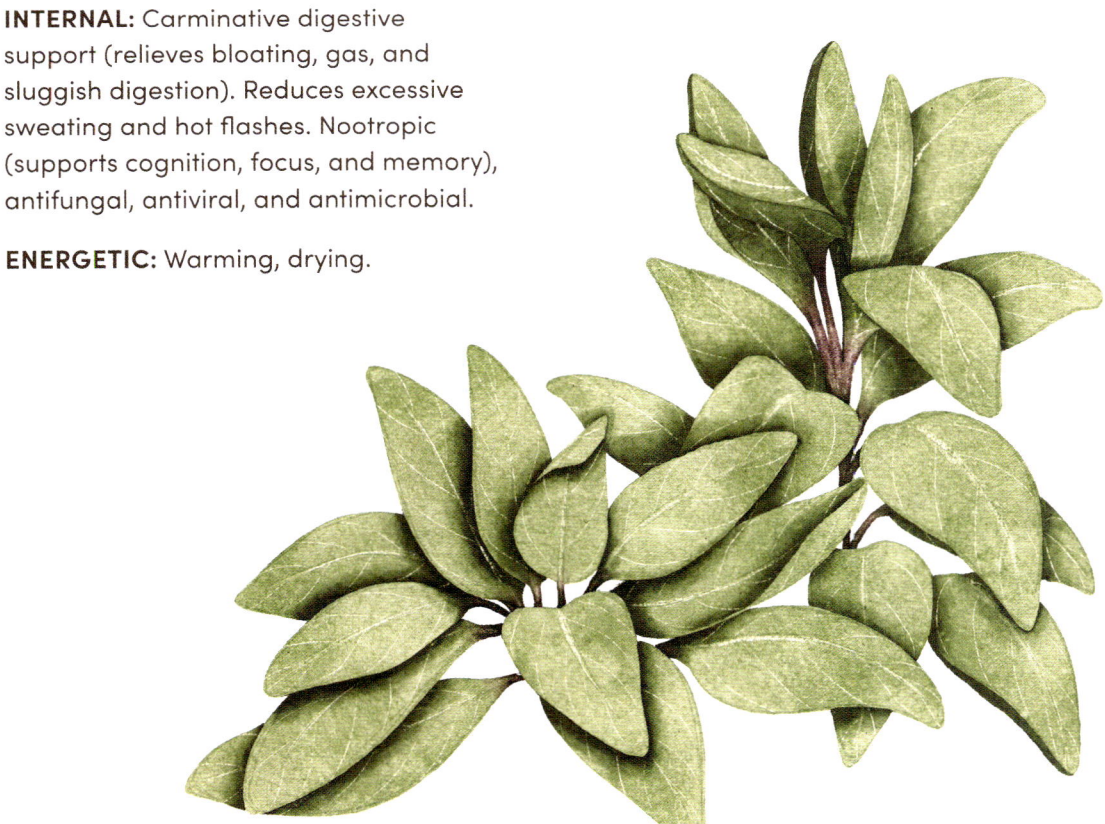

How to Grow:

 WHEN TO PLANT: Sow seeds indoors 6–8 weeks before the last frost, or transplant in spring once soil has warmed. In mild winter regions, sage can be transplanted in fall.

 GROWS BEST FROM: Transplants or stem cuttings. Seeds can be slow to germinate with variable success. Sow more seeds than you need to end up with enough successful sprouts. Sow seeds about ¼" deep and cover lightly with soil and mist with water. Germination can take at least 10–21 days. Stem cuttings root easily and produce stronger plants. Transplants give you a head start on the establishment of your sage.

 SUN AND SOIL NEEDS: Full sun, 6–8 hours or more. Needs well-draining, sandy, or loamy soil. Avoid heavy clay. Once established, sage is drought tolerant.

 VARIETIES TO TRY: Common sage, purple sage, tricolor sage, Berggarten sage, Greek sage, and white sage.

 SPACING: Space plants 18–24" apart. Sage forms a woody shrub up to 2' tall and wide, so give room for airflow to avoid fungal issues. Container friendly.

 BLOOM TIME: Typically 75–90 days from seed to leaf harvest. Transplants or cuttings take 60–75 days.

 HARVESTING TIPS: Begin cutting leaves once the plant is well established (6–8" tall). Harvest before or during bloom for the strongest flavor and medicinal oils. Regular cutting encourages bushier, more productive plants.

GOOD TO KNOW:

Sage has been treasured since ancient times as a sacred herb. Its botanical name, *Salvia*, derives from the Latin word *salvere*, meaning "to save" or "to heal." Ancient cultures, including the Romans, revered sage as a "holy herb," using it in sacred rituals and believing it granted longevity and improved memory.

How to Use:

 INFUSED OIL: Can be infused for antimicrobial salves, chest rubs, and topical healing.

 TINCTURE: 1 part fresh leaves to 2 parts 65–75% alcohol, or 1 part dried leaves to 5 parts 40–50% alcohol. Used to reduce sweating, alleviate anxiety, minimize excessive breast milk production, and boost memory.

 TEA: Steep 1–2 teaspoons dried leaves, or 1 tablespoon fresh leaves, per 1 cup hot water, covered, for 10–15 minutes. Sage tea can be used as a gargle for sore throats.

 POULTICE AND COMPRESS: Crushed fresh leaves can be applied as a poultice, or try a strong tea compress applied to inflamed skin or gums.

 General Safety:

TOPICAL USE: Generally well tolerated, though essential oil should be diluted because it can be irritating.

INTERNAL USE: Safe in culinary and tea doses. Avoid excessive amounts or long-term high doses due to potential nervous system effects, especially for those with seizure disorders. Pregnant and nursing women should avoid strong medicinal doses. Culinary use is fine. Sage can reduce milk supply, so nursing mothers should use caution.

HERBALIST TIP:

Sage is not only a flavorful kitchen staple but also used medicinally for menopause support. It contains essential oils and tannins that influence the nervous system and sweat regulation, which can help with hot flashes and night sweats, and memory-enhancing properties that can ease irritability.

Self-Heal

Prunella vulgaris
Perennial in zones 4–9

A hardy, low-growing member of the mint family, self-heal is known for its purple flower spikes and creeping habit. Traditionally called "heal-all" or "all-heal," self-heal has been valued for centuries as a wound remedy.

Medicinal Properties:

TOPICAL: Antimicrobial and astringent. Supports wound healing, insect bites, rashes, cuts, burns, and sore throats (when used in washes or poultices).

INTERNAL: Mild lymphatic. Supports immune balance, sore throats, fevers, digestive upset, and inflammation. Considered a gentle adaptogen.

ENERGETIC: Cooling, moistening.

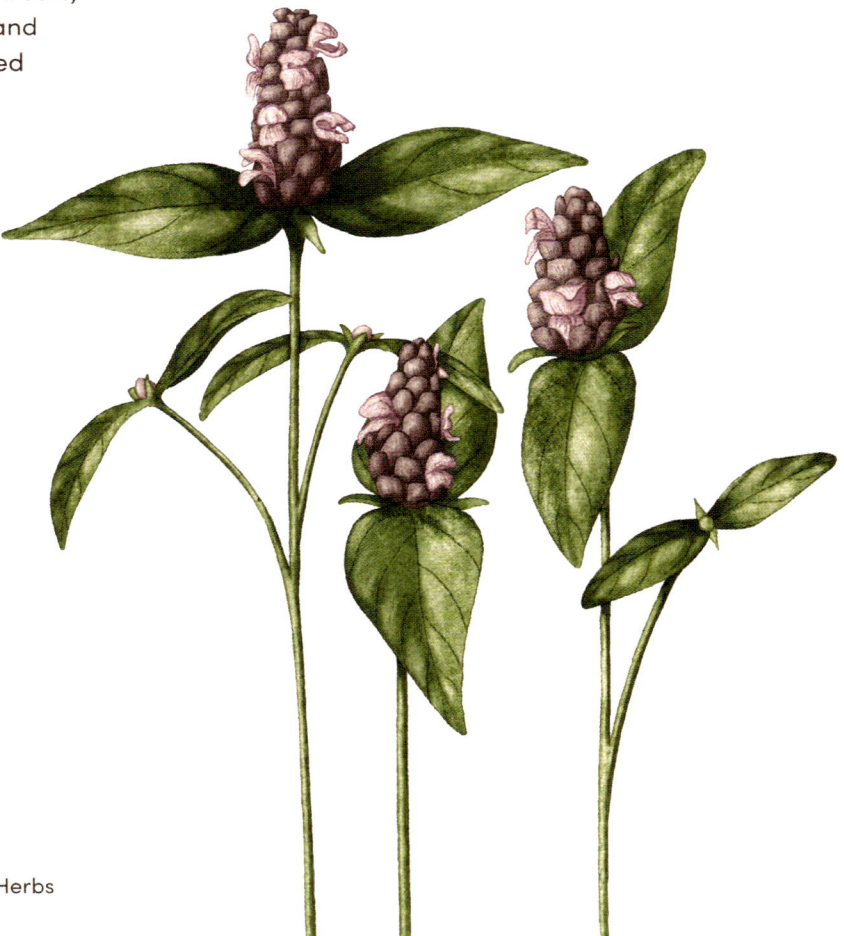

How to Grow:

 WHEN TO PLANT: Sow seeds outdoors in early spring or fall. In cooler climates, spring sowing works well. In warmer zones, fall sowing allows seedlings to establish before summer. You can also start seeds indoors 6–8 weeks before your last frost and transplant outside.

 GROWS BEST FROM: Seeds, but it's also easy to establish from root division or rooted cuttings. Plants spread by creeping rhizomes and can be dug up from established plants to divide and replant to get more plants. Self-heal is a slow starter, so expect 3–4 weeks for germination after cold stratification.

 SUN AND SOIL NEEDS: Prefers partial sun to light shade. Tolerates a range of soils but thrives in moist, well-drained soil with a bit of afternoon shade.

 VARIETIES TO TRY: *Prunella vulgaris* var. *lanceolata* and *Prunella grandiflora*.

 SPACING: Space plants 6–12" apart, as plants can spread outward by creeping roots. Container friendly.

 BLOOM TIME: 90–120 days from germination to first ight harvest of leaves, with peak flowering and medicinal potency in mid to late summer (June through August, depending on the zone).

 HARVESTING TIPS: Harvest young leaves in spring and early summer before flowering for best flavor and potency. Harvest flower spikes when about half of the blooms are open (midsummer). This ensures strong medicinal quality and continued flowering if harvested regularly.

GOOD TO KNOW:

Self-heal is edible; young leaves and flowers can be tossed into salads or soups. Self-heal also produces flowers that can attract pollinators.

How to Use:

 INFUSED OIL: Fresh or dried aerial parts (flowers, stems, and leaves) can be infused into oil for skin-healing salves.

 TINCTURE: 1 part fresh herb to 2 parts 70–95% alcohol, or 1 part dried herb to 5 parts 40% alcohol. Good for lymphatic and immune support.

 TEA: Steep 1–2 teaspoons dried herb, or 2–3 tablespoons fresh lightly crushed leaves, per 1 cup hot water for 10–15 minutes. Strong tea can be used as a gargle for sore throats, mouth ulcers, or gum irritation.

 POULTICE AND COMPRESS: Mashed fresh leaves can be applied as a poultice directly to wounds, or steeped as a tea and soaked into a compress to help with inflamed tissues.

 General Safety:

TOPICAL USE: Generally safe and well tolerated.

INTERNAL USE: Safe in normal tea or tincture doses for most people. Traditionally considered safe in moderate tea amounts for pregnant women. Avoid high-dose tincture without guidance.

HERBALIST TIP:

Self-heal is excellent combined with calendula or plantain leaf in wound-healing salves. Calendula adds antimicrobial strength, while plantain soothes and draws out irritation.

Skullcap

Scutellaria lateriflora

Perennial in zones 4–8

This is a delicate, leafy perennial in the mint family with small blue-violet flowers. Known as a powerful nervine herb, skullcap has long been valued for its ability to calm the nervous system.

Medicinal Properties:

TOPICAL: Not commonly used externally.

INTERNAL: Nervine tonic; reduces anxiety, quiets racing thoughts, and promotes restful sleep. Traditionally used for withdrawal support because of its nervous system–balancing effects. Supports restless leg issues and nervous digestive upset.

ENERGETIC: Cooling, drying.

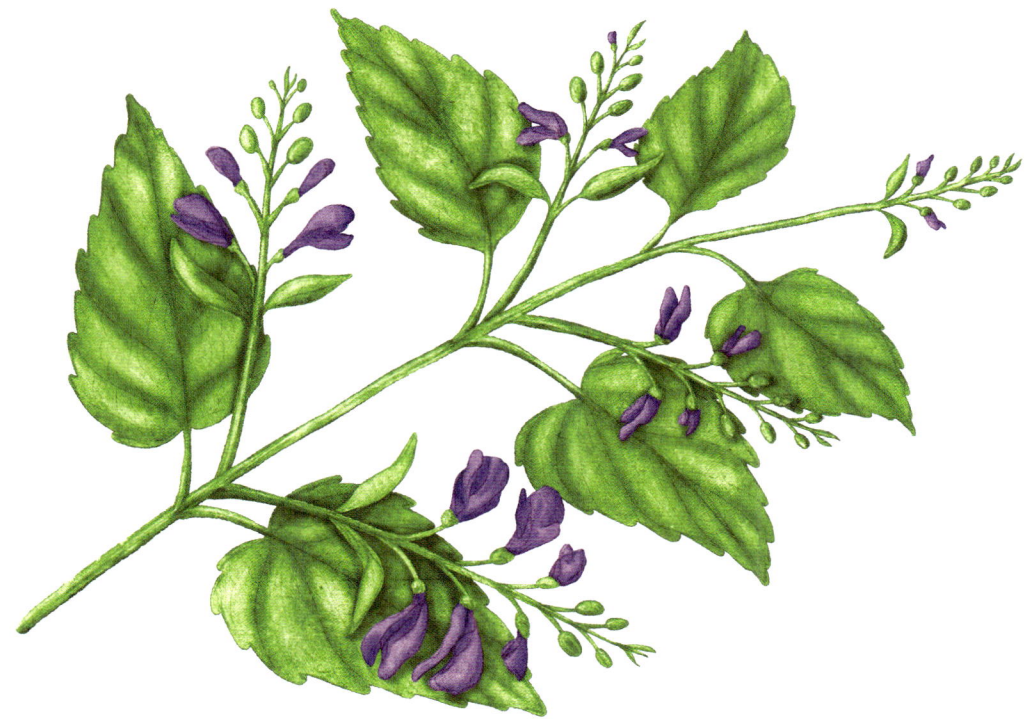

How to Grow:

 WHEN TO PLANT: Direct sow in late spring after the danger of frost has passed, or start indoors 6–8 weeks before last frost for transplanting.

 GROWS BEST FROM: Seed, root division, or stem cuttings. Seed germination can be slow, so dividing established clumps is a good option. Cold stratification improves germination. Seeds need light to germinate. Sow only on the surface of the soil and press in gently. Germination can take 10–20 days or longer.

 SUN AND SOIL NEEDS: Full sun to partial shade and well-drained soil. Tolerant of poorer soils but thrives with moderate fertility. Regular moisture is needed when establishing young plants. Once mature, semi-regular, deep waterings are preferred. In hotter climates, skullcap appreciates afternoon shade and moist, loamy soil that drains well, as it typically grows near stream banks and moist meadows. Mulching skullcap can help moderate moisture levels in summer months as well.

 VARIETIES TO TRY: American skullcap, Baikal skullcap, and heartleaf skullcap.

 SPACING: Space plants 12–18" apart. Skullcap tends to spread slowly by rhizomes, eventually forming small colonies.

 BLOOM TIME: 90–120 days from initial seeding to harvest. Start small harvests of leaves by mid to late summer of the first year. Establishes best in its second year, producing more vigorous foliage and flowers suitable for larger harvests.

 HARVESTING TIPS: Harvest aerial parts (flowers and leaves) just before or during flowering for best medicinal quality. Take light harvests only in the first year of growth so the plant can root in and return strong the following year.

GOOD TO KNOW:

Skullcap is different from Baikal skullcap (*Scutellaria baicalensis*), which is used more for immune and anti-inflammatory support in traditional Chinese medicine. Make sure you get the right species for your intended use.

How to Use:

 INFUSED OIL: Not typically used, but can be applied to temples for tension.

 TINCTURE: 1 part fresh aerial parts to 2 parts 50–60% alcohol, or 1 part dried aerial parts to 5 parts 40% alcohol. Fresh plant tinctures are considered most potent and are preferred. Used to reduce anxiety and overwhelm, racing thoughts, and insomnia. Can also help with tension headaches, tremors, spasms, and muscle tension.

 TEA: Steep 1–2 teaspoons dried herb, or 2 tablespoon fresh herb, per 1 cup hot water, covered, for 10–15 minutes. It is very bitter, so it's often blended with other herbs. Although alcohol is a better solvent for extracting the medicinal properties of skullcap, tea made with this herb can provide gentle calming benefits for those with anxiety, burnout, and insomnia.

 POULTICE AND COMPRESS: A poultice or compress can be applied to temples or forehead for stress headaches.

General Safety:

TOPICAL USE: Generally safe, though rarely used externally.

INTERNAL USE: Generally well tolerated, though large doses may cause drowsiness. Limited data exists for pregnant or nursing women.

HERBALIST TIP:

Skullcap works best when taken consistently over time, rather than as a one-time dose. Think of it as a tonic for rebuilding an exhausted nervous system, especially in cases of chronic stress, overwork, or long-standing anxiety.

Stevia

Stevia rebaudiana
Perennial in zones 9–11

A leafy green plant native to South America, stevia is prized for its intensely sweet leaves that contain natural compounds called steviol glycosides, which are two hundred to three hundred times sweeter than sugar, but without the calories.

Medicinal Properties:

TOPICAL: Not commonly used externally.

INTERNAL: Widely used as a natural noncaloric sweetener. Supports healthy blood sugar balance and oral health.

ENERGETIC:
Cooling, drying.

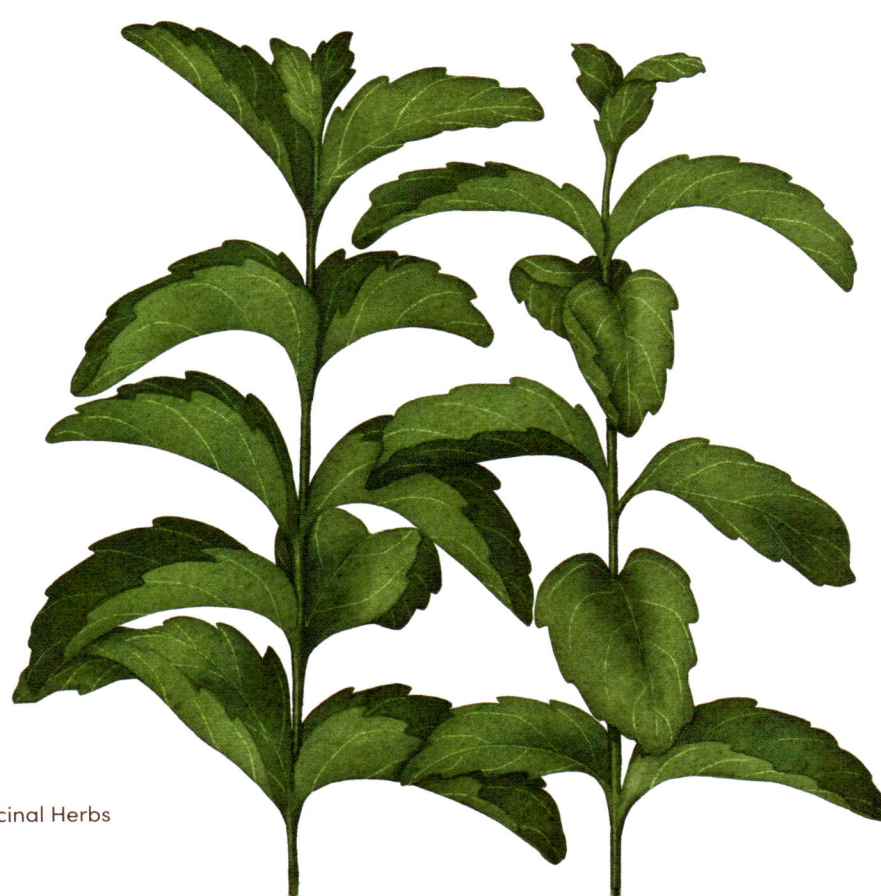

How to Grow:

 WHEN TO PLANT: Direct sow in spring after the danger of frost has passed, or start indoors 6–8 weeks before last frost.

 GROWS BEST FROM: Seed or transplant. Seeds need light to germinate, so press into the soil surface rather than covering. Germination takes 10–14 days. It can also self-seed once established.

 SUN AND SOIL NEEDS: Full sun, 6–8 hours or more, and well-drained soil. Stevia does not like "wet feet" or heavy clay soil. Stevia does better with soil pH in the 6.0–6.5 range, so it can struggle in alkaline soils. Adding compost or peat moss can help amend the soil. Too much nitrogen (from animal-based compost or blood meal) can make lush growth, but will reduce leaf sweetness. Regular moisture is needed when establishing young plants. Once mature, regular, deep waterings are preferred.

 VARIETIES TO TRY: Criolla, Morita II, and commercial hybrids.

 SPACING: Space plants 12–18" apart to allow airflow and prevent mildew. Stevia can get up to 2' tall and is bushy in shape. Container friendly.

 BLOOM TIME: Typically 90–120 days from seed and 60–90 days from transplants.

 HARVESTING TIPS: Harvest young leaves throughout the growing season, pinching stems to encourage branching. For the sweetest leaves, collect in late summer just before flowering.

GROWING TIP:

Stevia leaves are sweetest just before flowering. Pinching off flower buds will prolong leaf sweetness and leaf production. In colder climates, stevia is best grown as an annual or overwintered indoors in pots.

How to Use:

To Make Stevia Extract: To make a liquid extract of stevia sweetener, pack 1 cup freshly chopped leaves into a jar covered with 40–50% alcohol. Vodka is best for this. Cap and store in a dark place for 24–48 hours; don't exceed, to avoid bitterness. Strain and let liquid sit out in a well ventilated area, stirring occasionally until alcohol vapors dissipate. Store in a dropper bottle for 3–6 months. For an alcohol-free extract, add 1 cup fresh leaves, or ½ cup dried leaves, to 1½ cups vegetable glycerin. Jar per previous extract instructions. Steep for 2–4 weeks and strain. Store in a dropper bottle in the fridge for about 6 months.

 INFUSED OIL: Not typically made with this herb.

 TINCTURE: Not typically made with this herb.

 TEA: Typically used as a sweetener, not a standalone tea. Add a few fresh leaves to your cup of herbal tea for a slight addition of sweetness. Or, add ⅛ teaspoon ground stevia leaves to 1–2 teaspoons herbal tea blend before steeping.

 POULTICE AND COMPRESS: Not typically used as a poultice or compress.

General Safety:

TOPICAL USE: Generally safe, though rarely used externally.

INTERNAL USE: Considered safe for most people in culinary amounts. High doses of concentrated extract may cause digestive upset in sensitive individuals. Culinary amounts are considered safe for pregnant and nursing women, but concentrated extract is best avoided unless under guidance. Those who are trying to get pregnant should avoid stevia extract, as it has been shown to have some mild contraceptive effects that may impact fertility during use.

HERBALIST TIP:

Stevia can be known for its bitterness when concentrated too far. If you are sensitive to the bitterness of this herb, consider adding just a couple of smashed leaves into your teas to gently sweeten them. Unlike sugar, stevia does not feed yeast or contribute to candida overgrowth, making it popular among those on low-sugar diets. Dried and ground stevia powder can be used in baking recipes, but it will carry a slight green color from its raw state.

St.-John's-Wort

Hypericum perforatum
Perennial in zones 5–10

This bright, sun-loving herb has clusters of yellow star-shaped flowers that release a red pigment when crushed. It has long been valued as a nervous system tonic and topical wound healer.

Medicinal Properties:

TOPICAL: Antimicrobial that is soothing to nerve pain, burns, bruises, muscle aches, and minor wounds.

INTERNAL: Mild antidepressant and nervous system tonic that treats anxiety, seasonal affective disorder, nerve pain, and recovery after stress or trauma.

ENERGETIC: Cooling, drying.

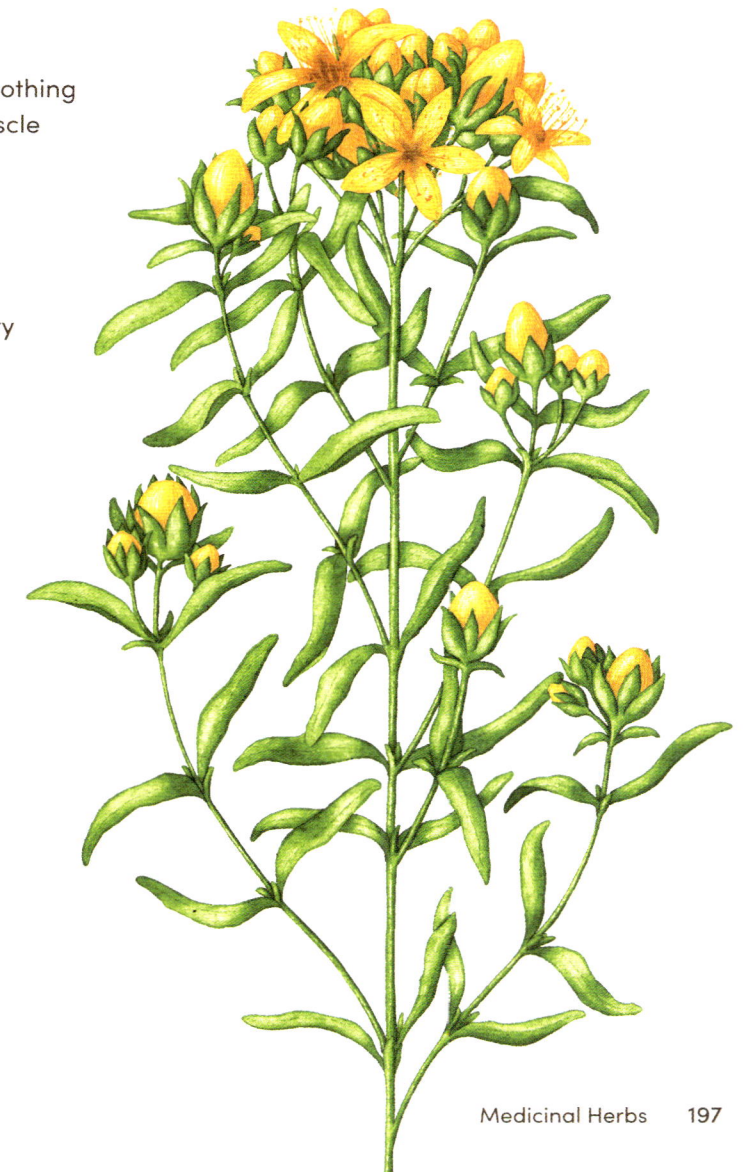

How to Grow:

 WHEN TO PLANT: Start seeds indoors 8–10 weeks before your last frost, or transplant propagated root divisions, cuttings, or live plants in spring once the ground has warmed in colder winter climates (zones 5–7) or in the early fall in warmer winter climates (zones 8–11).

 GROWS BEST FROM: Transplant or root division. Seeds are tiny and slow to germinate. They require light to germinate, so press seeds onto the soil surface without covering. St.-John's-wort grows by rhizomatous roots that can be dug up in clumps and divided to replant in other areas as propagations. Cuttings can be taken from soft stems in late spring/early summer and rooted in water and replanted to grow more plants as well.

 SUN AND SOIL NEEDS: Full sun, 6–8 hours or more, and well-draining sandy or rocky soil. Tolerates poor soil but thrives in moderate fertility. Drought tolerant once established.

 VARIETIES TO TRY: *Hypericum perforatum, Hypericum calycinum,* and *Hypericum olympicum.*

 SPACING: Space plants 18–24" apart. Grows as a shrubby perennial that can get anywhere from 1–3' tall and 1–2' wide. Container friendly.

 BLOOM TIME: In the first year, plants stay relatively small and may not bloom until late in the season, sometimes producing only a handful of flowers. Stronger flowering occurs 1 year or more after seeding, once the plant is established. Established plants transplanted in spring can produce flowers the same summer, typically 90–120 days after transplanting.

 HARVESTING TIPS: Harvest when flowers are just opening, as this is when hypericin and hyperforin are most concentrated. The aerial parts (flowers, stems, and leaves) should be cut during peak bloom.

GOOD TO KNOW:

St.-John's-wort contains hypericin and hyperforin, compounds that support mood. The infused oil made with this herb is one of the best remedies for nerve-related pain.

How to Use:

 INFUSED OIL: Fresh flowers can be infused into oils, salves, and balms for use with burns, sore muscles, and nerve pain.

 TINCTURE: 1 part aerial parts (flowers, stems, and leaves) to 2 parts 70–80% alcohol, or 1 part aerial parts to 5 parts 40–50% alcohol. The fresh flowers of St.-John's-wort contain the highest concentration of medicinal properties. Used for mood support and easing anxiety and mild depression.

 TEA: Steep 1–2 teaspoons dried aerial parts, or 1 tablespoon fresh aerial parts, per 1 cup hot water, covered, for 10 minutes. Tea is a less common preparation for St.-John's-wort due to bitterness, but it can be used for mild depression or anxiety.

 POULTICE AND COMPRESS: Crushed fresh flowers can be applied as a poultice externally for helping heal wounds, bruises, or burns. A warm compress can be made with St.-John's-wort to ease nerve pain and muscle cramps. A cooled compress can be helpful to reduce swelling and heal damaged tissues.

⚠ General Safety:

TOPICAL USE: Well tolerated by most people, but may cause mild photosensitivity in very light-skinned individuals when applied topically followed by prolonged sun exposure.

INTERNAL USE: Can cause photosensitivity in some people. Most importantly, St.-John's-wort interacts with many medications (antidepressants, birth control pills, blood thinners, and HIV and cancer drugs) by speeding their breakdown in the liver. Should be used with professional guidance. Pregnant and nursing women should avoid internal use due to limited safety data.

HERBALIST TIP:

For maximum potency, harvest flowers on a sunny day just as they open and immediately begin an oil or tincture. Waiting even a few hours can reduce their medicinal strength. The red color in the oil or tincture is your sign that the medicine is strong.

Thyme

Thymus vulgaris

Perennial in zones 5–9 (some creeping varieties hardy to zone 4)

This low-growing, woody-stemmed perennial herb with tiny, aromatic leaves and delicate clusters of purple, pink, or white flowers (which bloom in the summer) is loved by pollinators. Thyme adds flavor to the kitchen and has long been valued for its medicinal and preservative qualities.

Medicinal Properties:

TOPICAL: Antiseptic and antifungal. Helps with skin infections and minor wounds.

INTERNAL: Carminative, expectorant, and antimicrobial. Helps relieve coughs, sore throat, bronchitis, gas, and indigestion.

ENERGETIC: Warming, drying.

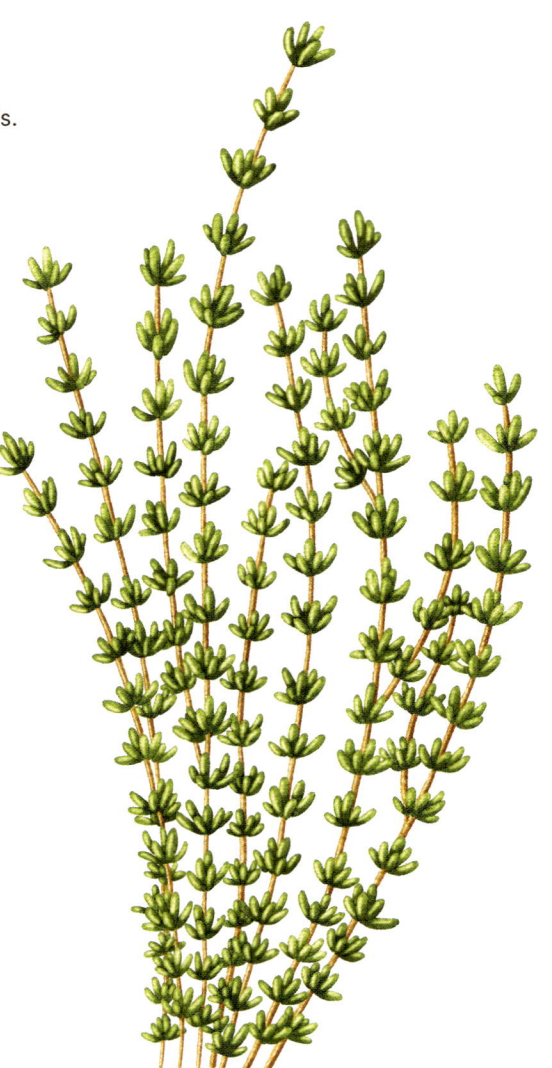

HERBALIST TIP:

Thyme tea is especially effective when taken at the first sign of a cough or sore throat to help prevent the infection from settling deeper into the lungs.

How to Grow:

 WHEN TO PLANT: Sow seeds indoors 6–10 weeks before last frost or transplant live plants once soil has warmed.

 GROWS BEST FROM: Transplants, root division, or cuttings, as seeds are very slow and can be finicky. Seeds need light to germinate and can take 14–28 days to sprout. Sprinkle seeds on the surface of soil and keep moist. Softwood cuttings root easily in spring and summer. Once plants are established, you can divide chunks of the root system by digging them up and replanting them elsewhere to get more plants.

 SUN AND SOIL NEEDS: Full sun, 6–8 hours or more. Prefers well-draining sandy or rocky soil with low fertility. Overly rich soil will reduce aromatic oils.

 VARIETIES TO TRY: Common thyme, French thyme, lemon thyme, lime thyme, woolly thyme, creeping thyme, German thyme, English thyme, Doone Valley, and Archer's Gold.

 SPACING: Space plants 12–18" apart for upright thyme. Creeping types can be planted closer to 6–12" apart to create ground cover or fill in gaps between stones. Container friendly.

 BLOOM TIME: Typically 150–180 days from seed to leaf harvest and 60–90 days from transplants or cuttings until first harvest of leaves.

 HARVESTING TIPS: Cut stems back just above a leaf node to encourage bushy regrowth. Harvest in the morning, after the dew has dried but before the sun is too hot. This is when essential oil concentration is highest.

GROWING TIP:

Thyme contains thymol, a powerful antimicrobial compound used in natural cleaning and oral care products. The plant thrives in tough conditions with little care, making it a favorite for rock gardens, pathways, and herb spirals. Overwatering is the quickest way to kill thyme.

How to Use:

 INFUSED OIL: Dried thyme can be infused to be used as an antiseptic and antifungal oil for salves and skin infections.

 TINCTURE: 1 part fresh thyme leaves to 2 parts 70–90% alcohol, or 1 part dried thyme leaves to 5 parts 40–50% alcohol. Used as a powerful antimicrobial, a deep expectorant, a cough suppressant (making coughs more effective but less frequent and spasmodic), an intestinal antiseptic, a carminative to relieve gas and bloating, and a circulatory stimulant.

 TEA: Steep 1–2 teaspoons dried leaves, or 1 tablespoon fresh leaves, per 1 cup hot water for 10–15 minutes. Used for suppressing a cough, relieving a sore throat, boosting immunity, relieving gas and bloating, and easing cramps.

 POULTICE AND COMPRESS: Crushed fresh leaves can be made into a poultice or tea-soaked compress and applied to the chest for coughs or minor skin issues.

 STEAM INHALATION: Add a handful of fresh thyme to hot water. Tent your head with a towel and inhale for 5–10 minutes for bronchial support. This is one of the most widely used methods for utilizing the benefits of thyme.

⚠ General Safety:

TOPICAL USE: Generally safe, but concentrated essential oil may cause irritation and should be diluted.

INTERNAL USE: Safe in culinary and tea amounts for most people. Avoid strong tinctures in high doses during pregnancy.

Turmeric

Curcuma longa
Perennial in zones 8–12

This tropical clumping perennial from the ginger family, with lush canna lily–like leaves and underground orange rhizomes, is prized for its culinary spice and potent anti-inflammatory uses.

Medicinal Properties:

TOPICAL: Helps with bruises, inflammation, and joint pain.

INTERNAL: Potent anti-inflammatory and blood purifier. Stimulates bile production to support a sluggish liver and improve constipation. Improves mood and circulation.

ENERGETIC: Warming, slightly drying.

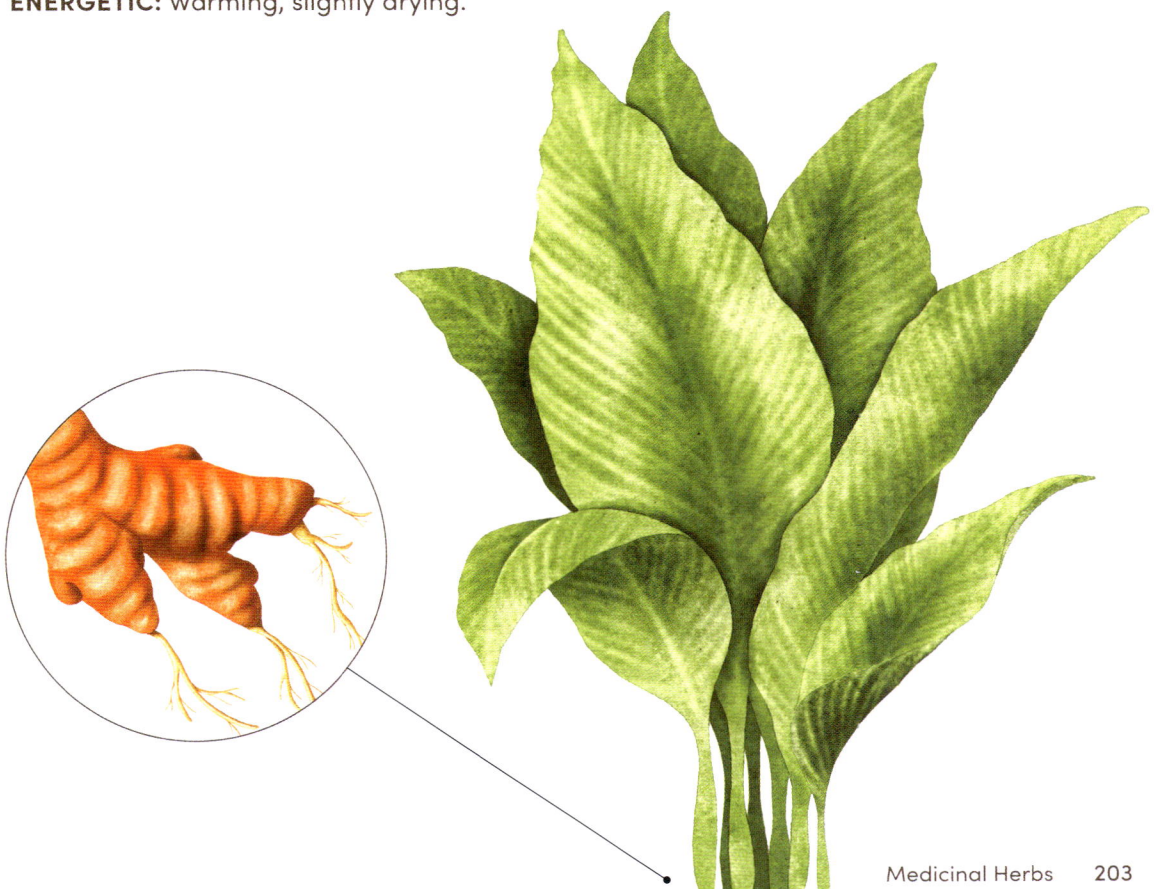

How to Grow:

 WHEN TO PLANT: Plant turmeric rhizomes directly outdoors once soil temps are consistently above 60°F, after the threat of last frost has passed. In tropical areas, turmeric can be planted year-round. In colder climates, you can start sprouting the rhizomes inside under grow lights to transplant outside when nights are warmer.

 GROWS BEST FROM: Rhizome. You can sprout or directly sow with at least one bud (which is where the sprouts form). These can be dug up and divided each year to make more plants.

 SUN AND SOIL NEEDS: Partial shade to filtered sun. In very hot climates, turmeric does best with afternoon shade or dappled light to prevent scorching. It needs loose, rich, loamy soil that drains well. Turmeric does not like compacted, heavy clay soils, and rhizomes will rot if waterlogged. Dry soil slows rhizome development.

 VARIETIES TO TRY: Indian turmeric, Hawaiian turmeric, and Thai turmeric.

 SPACING: Sow rhizomes 8–12" apart, or 12–18" apart if planting in rows. Plant rhizomes 2–4" deep with the buds' "eyes" facing upward. Containers should be at least 12" wide per plant. Wide, shallow containers are best for rhizomes, because they spread horizontally.

 BLOOM TIME: Baby turmeric (the young, pale rhizomes) are usually ready 4–5 months after planting. Fully mature turmeric need 8–10 months of warm weather after planting.

 HARVESTING TIPS: Harvest rhizomes when leaves start yellowing and dying back in late fall. Save some rhizomes to dry and store for replanting in the spring.

HERBALIST TIP:

Turmeric is best used consistently in small daily amounts rather than in occasional large doses. "Golden milk" is a common turmeric tea recipe that is used to help the curcumin compound in turmeric become the most bioavailable to the body by incorporating the fat from milk and a pinch of black pepper to maximize the potency of this herb. Consider adding milk or a fat to your turmeric tea for extra effectiveness.